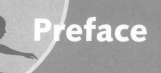

Preface

Anatomy has been taught as a discipline for over 2000 years, and current health affairs students join the legions of those preceding them in having to learn a new language, master comprehension of difficult three-dimensional relationships, and understand the intricacies of the many different tissue and organ systems that comprise the wonderful machine that is the human body. In the information age, the time available to do this is often limited by the number and content of the other areas of knowledge needed to practice modern medicine.

The first American edition of *Crash Course: Anatomy* is designed to help students handle this daunting task, with a concise presentation of the overall material, including mnemonics, figures, and clinical information for each region of the body. Summaries of what a student should learn from each chapter reinforce the material. This book contains sufficient detail to provide a useful review before exams for students in medicine, dentistry, and allied health professions; it is especially relevant for the USMLE Part I. It also provides a good review of basic anatomic knowledge needed by students doing clerkships in the individual disciplines of surgery, orthopedics, obstetrics and gynecology, otolaryngology, and radiology.

To all of the students who use this book, I wish you good luck in your studies and a bright future in medicine!

Noelle A. Granger

CRASH COURSE
Anatomy

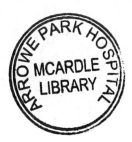
This book is due for return on or before the last date shown below.

Other titles in the Crash Course series

There are 23 books in the Crash Course series in two ranges: Basic Science and Clinical. Each book follows the same format, with concise text, clear illustrations and helpful learning features including access to online USMLE test questions.

Basic Science titles
Pathology
Nervous System
Renal and Urinary Systems
Gastrointestinal System
Respiratory System
Endocrine and Reproductive Systems
Metabolism and Nutrition
Pharmacology
Immunology
Musculoskeletal System
Cardiovascular System
Cell Biology and Genetics
Anatomy

Clinical titles
Surgery
Cardiology
History and Examination
Internal Medicine
Neurology
Gastroenterology
OBGYN

Forthcoming:
Pyschiatry
Imaging
Pediatrics

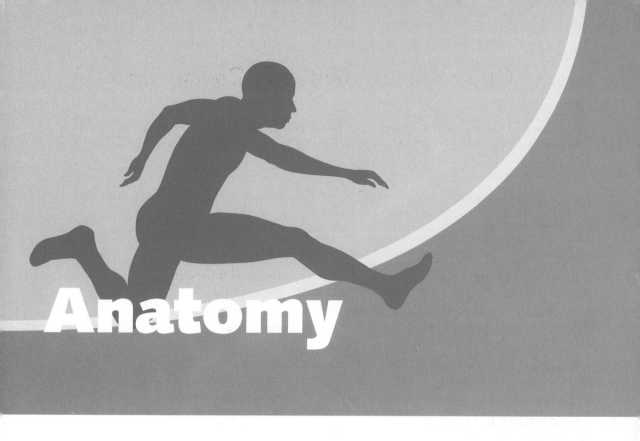

Anatomy

Noelle A. Granger, PhD

Professor, Department of Cell and Developmental Biology
University of North Carolina School of Medicine
Chapel Hill, North Carolina

UK edition authors
Michael Dykes, Phillip Ameerally

UK series editor
Daniel Horton-Szar

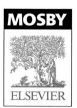

MOSBY

ELSEVIER

1600 John F. Kennedy Blvd.
Suite 1800
Philadelphia, PA 19103-2899

CRASH COURSE: ANATOMY
Copyright ©2007 by Mosby, Inc., an affiliate of Elsevier, Inc.

ISBN-13: 978-0-323-04319-9
ISBN-10: 0-323-04319-4

Notice

Knowledge and best practice in this field are constantly changing. As new research and experience broaden our knowledge, changes in practice, treatment and drug therapy may become necessary or appropriate. Readers are advised to check the most current information provided (i) on procedures featured or (ii) by the manufacturer of each product to be administered, to verify the recommended dose or formula, the method and duration of administration, and contraindications. It is the responsibility of the practitioner, relying on their own experience and knowledge of the patient, to make diagnoses, to determine dosages and the best treatment for each individual patient, and to take all appropriate safety precautions. To the fullest extant of the law, neither the Publisher nor the Author assumes any liability for any injury and/or damage to persons or property arising out of or related to any use of the material contained in this book.

The Publisher

Adapted from Crash Course: Anatomy, 2e by Michael Dykes and Phillip Ameerally, ISBN: 0-7234-3247-3. © 2002, Elsevier Science Limited.

The rights of Michael Dykes and Phillip Ameerally to be identified as the authors of this book have been asserted in accordance with the Copyright, Designs and Patents Act, 1988.

Library of Congress Cataloging-in-Publication Data

Granger, Noelle (Noelle A.)
   Crash course anatomy / Noelle Granger.—1st American ed.
      p. cm.
   Includes index.
   ISBN 0-323-04319-4
   1. Human anatomy.   I. Title
   QM23.2.G673 2007
   611—dc22

2006046220

Acquisitions Editor: Alex Stibbe
Project Development Manager: Stan Ward
Publishing Services Manager: David Saltzberg
Designer: Andy Chapman
Cover Design: Antbits Illustration
Illustration Manager: Mick Ruddy

Printed in China

Last digit is the print number:
9 8 7 6 5 4 3 2 1

Acknowledgments

I would like to thank the authors of the first and second UK editions, Michael Dykes and Phillip Ameerally, for creating an excellent structural framework. Their understanding of an anatomic core of knowledge is exceptional.

Dedication

To my husband, R. Eugene Granger, MD, for his constant patience and support during my work on this book, and to two of the classical anatomists, O.W. Henson and William Pollitzer, who taught me anatomy and who taught humanity as well.

Contents

1. Basic Concepts of Anatomy

Descriptive anatomic terms

The anatomic position

This is a standard position used in anatomy and clinical medicine to allow accurate and consistent description of one body part in relation to another (Fig. 1.1):

- The head is directed forwards with eyes looking into the distance.
- The body is upright, legs together, and directed forwards.
- The palms are turned forward, with the thumbs laterally.

Regions of the body

Regions of the body are shown in Fig. 1.1. Note that the upper limb is composed of the scapular region, the arm, the forearm, and the hand; the lower limb is composed of the gluteal region, the thigh, the leg, and the foot.

Anatomic planes

These comprise the following (Fig. 1.2):

- The median sagittal plane is the vertical plane passing through the midline of the body, dividing it into right and left halves. Any plane parallel to this is termed paramedian or sagittal.
- Coronal (or frontal) planes are vertical planes, dividing the body into anterior (front) and posterior (back) segments.
- Horizontal or transverse planes pass through the body from front to back, dividing it into superior (upper) and inferior (lower) segments.

Terms of position

The terms of position commonly used in clinical practice and anatomy are illustrated in Fig. 1.3.

Terms of movement

Various terms are used to describe movements of the body (Fig. 1.4):

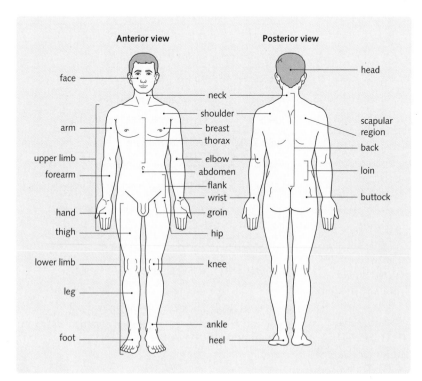

Fig. 1.1 Anatomic position and regions of the body.

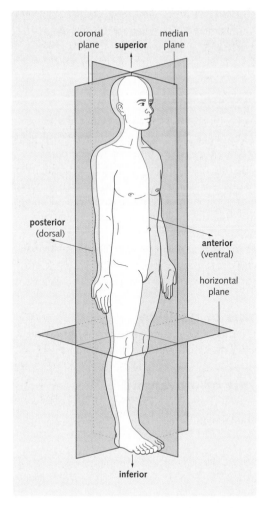

Fig. 1.2 Anatomic planes.

- Flexion—movement that decreases the angle between the bones at a joint or between parts of the body, i.e., bending at the knee or elbow. *Dorsiflexion* describes flexion at the ankle such as when walking uphill, while *plantarflexion* describes flexion at the ankle that occurs when you stand on your toes.
- Extension—movement that increases the angle between the bones at a joint or between body parts, i.e, straightening the leg at the knee.
- Abduction—movement away from the median plane.
- Adduction—movement towards the median plane.
- Supination—movement, e.g., lateral rotation of the forearm, causing the palm to face anteriorly.

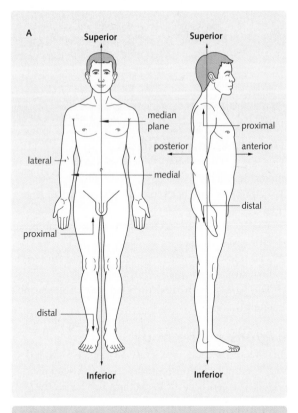

B	Classification of terms commonly used in anatomy and clinical practice	
Position	**Description**
Anterior	In front of another structure
Posterior	Behind another structure
Superior	Above another structure
Inferior	Below another structure
Deep	Farther away from body surface
Superficial	Close to body surface
Medial	Closer to median plane
Lateral	Farther away from medial plane
Proximal	Closer to the trunk or origin
Distal	Further away from the trunk or origin
Ipsilateral	The same side of the body
Contralateral	The opposite side of the body

Fig. 1.3 Relationship and comparison (A) and classification (B) of terms of position commonly used in anatomy and clinical practice.

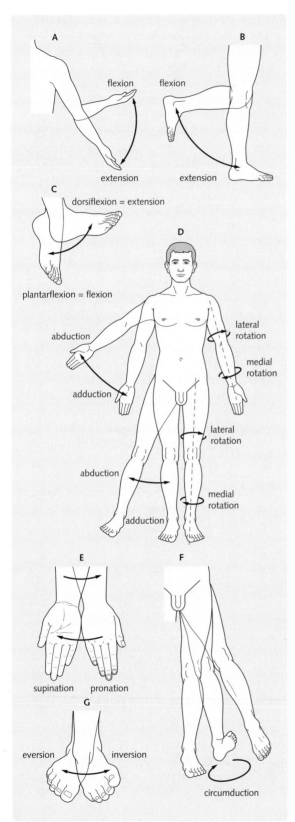

- Pronation—movement, e.g., medial rotation of the forearm, causing the palm to face posteriorly.
- Eversion—turning the sole of the foot outwards.
- Inversion—turning the sole of the foot inwards.
- Rotation—movement of part of the body around its longitudinal axis, i.e., turning one's head to the side.
- Circumduction—a combination of flexion, extension, abduction, and adduction so that the rotation of the distal end of a body part makes a circle.

The terms used to describe movements of the thumb are perpendicular to the movements of the body (Fig. 1.5).

To differentiate supination from pronation, remember that you hold a bowl of soup in the palm of your hand with a supinated forearm, but spill it if you pronate!

Basic structures of anatomy

Integument

The skin or integument is a good indicator of general health and is the largest organ of the body. The functions of the skin include:

- Protection from ultraviolet light, invading microorganisms, and mechanical, chemical, and thermal insults.
- Sensations including pain, temperature, touch, and pressure.
- Thermoregulation.
- Metabolic functions, e.g., vitamin D synthesis.

Fig. 1.4 Terms of movement. (A) Flexion and extension of forearm at elbow joint. (B) Flexion and extension of leg at knee joint. (C) Dorsiflexion and plantarflexion of foot at ankle joint. (D) Abduction and adduction of right limbs and rotation of left limbs at shoulder and hip joints, respectively. (E) Pronation and supination of forearm at radioulnar joints. (F) Circumduction (circular movement) of lower limb at hip joint. (G) Inversion and eversion of foot at subtalar and transverse tarsal joints.

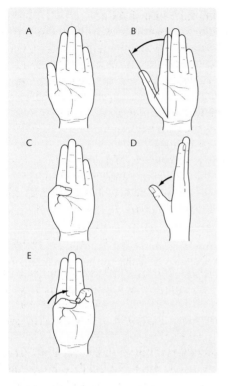

Fig. 1.5 Terms of movement for the thumb.
(A) Neutral hand position. (B) Extension. (C) Flexion.
(D) Abduction. (E) Opposition. (Adapted from Biswas
SV, Iqbal R: Crash Course: Musculoskeletal System.
St. Louis, Mosby.)

The skin is composed of the following (Fig. 1.6):
- The epidermis. This forms a protective
  waterproof barrier. It consists of a keratinized
  epithelium, a tough superficial layer that is
  continuously being shed, and a basal layer that
  is regenerative and pigmented. The epidermis is
  avascular and contains no lymphatics.
- The dermis. This supports the epidermis and
  has a rich network of vessels, afferent nerve
  endings, lymphatics, and hair follicles with
  their associated arrector pili muscles and
  sebaceous glands. It is composed mainly of
  collagen fibers with elastic fibers, giving the skin
  its elasticity.
- The hypodermis or superficial fascia. (See
  below.)

The skin appendages include:
- Hairs—highly modified, keratinized filaments
  arising from hair follicles in the dermis or
  superficial fascia.
- Sweat glands—single, coiled tubular glands in
  the dermis or superficial fascia that produce
  sweat, which plays a role in thermoregulation.
- Sebaceous glands—lobular glands that are
  appendages of hair follicles in the dermis or
  superficial fascia, which produce sebum, a wax-
  like, oily substance that lubricates the skin and
  hair.
- Nails—keratinized epithelial cells arranged in
  hard plates that develop in the dermis and that
  are found on the dorsal surface of each digit,
  i.e., finger or toe.

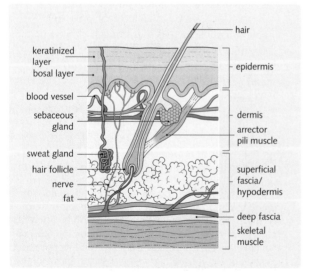

Fig. 1.6 Structure of skin and subcutaneous tissue.

Fascia

The fascia of the body may be divided into superficial and deep layers.

Superficial fascia (subcutaneous tissue) is composed of loose connective tissue, stored fat, sweat glands, blood vessels, lymphatic vessels, cutaneous nerves, and the roots of hair follicles and their associated arrector pili muscles.

In some places sheets of muscle lie in this fascia, e.g., muscles of facial expression.

The deep fascia is an organized connective tissue layer, deep to the superficial fascia, that surrounds the limbs and body. Extensions from the deep fascia surround individual muscles and neurovascular bundles, and intermuscular septa extend from the deep fascia, attach to bone, and divide limb musculature into compartments. This fascia contains no fat but has a rich nerve supply and is, therefore, very sensitive. The thickness of the fascia varies widely: e.g., it is thickened in the iliotibial tract but very thin over the rectus abdominis muscle and absent over the face. The arrangements of the compartments created by this fascia determine the pattern of spread of infection.

Bone

Bone is a specialized form of connective tissue with a mineralized extracellular matrix, within which bone cells are located. The functions of bone include:

- Structural framework for support and protection of body organs.
- Locomotion (by serving as a rigid lever).
- Calcium homeostasis and storage of other inorganic ions.
- Synthesis of blood cells.

Classification of bone

Bones are classified according to their location and shape. Their location can be within:

- Axial skeleton, e.g., skull, vertebral column including the sacrum, ribs, and sternum.
- Appendicular skeleton, e.g., hip bones, pectoral girdle, and bones of the upper and lower limbs.

Bones can be classified by their anatomic shape:

- Long bones, e.g., femur, humerus.
- Short bones, e.g., carpal bones.
- Flat bones, e.g., skull vault.
- Irregular bones, e.g., vertebrae.
- Sesamoid (bean-shaped) bones, e.g., the patella.

General structure of bone

Bone is surrounded by a connective tissue layer called the periosteum (Fig. 1.7), except where articular cartilage occurs at joints. The periosteum is vascular and provides the underlying bone with nutrients. It also contains progenitor cells and thus is capable of laying down more bone, and it provides the interface for the attachment of ligaments and tendons.

After a fracture, the fibroblast cells of the periosteum proliferate and secrete collagen, forming a cuff around the fracture site called a callus. The callus holds the fracture ends together and eventually is resorbed and replaced by bone.

In addition to the periosteum, bone includes the following components:

- An outer dense layer called compact or cortical bone that provides great strength and rigidity.
- A layer of cancellous or spongy bone that consists of a network of trabeculae arranged to resist external forces.
- A medullary cavity in long bones continuous with the interstices of cancellous bone, filled with red (hematopoietic) or yellow (fatty) marrow. At birth virtually all the bone marrow

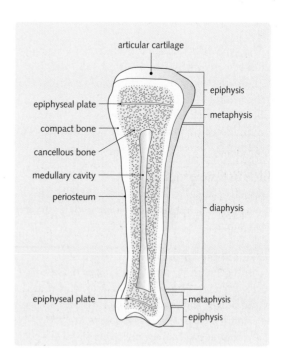

Fig. 1.7 Long bone and its components.

is red, but this is replaced by yellow marrow—
only the ribs, sternum, vertebrae, clavicle,
pelvis, and skull bones contain red marrow in
adult life.
- A single-cellular osteogenic layer called the
endosteum that lines the marrow cavity.

Blood supply of bones
There are two main sources of blood supply to
bone:
- A major nutrient artery that supplies the
marrow.
- Vessels from the periosteum.

The periosteal supply to bone assumes greater
importance in the elderly. Extensive stripping of
the periosteum, e.g., during surgery or following
trauma, may result in bone death.

Joints
These are unions between bones (Fig. 1.8).

Synovial joints
These have the following features:
- The bone ends are covered by hyaline articular
cartilage.
- The joint is surrounded by a joint capsule
consisting of a fibrous outer layer lined by a
serous synovial membrane, which does not
extend over the articular cartilage at the end of
the bones.
- The synovial membrane produces the synovial
fluid found within the joint capsule, which
lubricates the joint and transports nutrients to
the articular cartilage.
- Some synovial joints, e.g., the
temporomandibular joints, are divided into two
cavities by an articular disc.

Blood supply of joints
A vascular plexus of articular arteries from vessels
around the joint provides the joint with a very good
blood supply.

Nerve supply of joints
According to Hilton's law, the motor nerve to a
muscle tends to give a branch to the joint that the
muscle moves and another branch to the skin over
the joint. The capsule and ligaments are supplied
by afferent nerve endings including proprioceptive
and pain fibers. The synovial membrane contains
few pain fibers, and there are no afferent fibers in

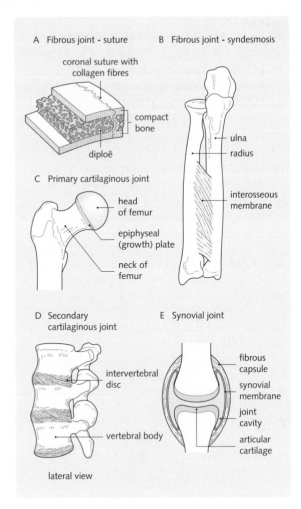

Fig. 1.8 Types of joints. (A) Fibrous joint—sutural
(bones are united by fibrous tissue, as in sutures of the
skull). (B) Fibrous joint—syndesmosis (bones are joined
by a sheet of fibrous tissue). (C) Primary cartilaginous
joint (where bone and hyaline cartilage meet). (D)
Secondary cartilaginous joint (articular surfaces are
covered by a thin lamina of hyaline cartilage; the
hyaline laminae are united by fibrocartilage). (E)
Synovial joint.

articular cartilage; joint pain is, therefore, localized
to the joint capsule and associated ligaments.

Stability of joints
Stability is achieved by the following components:
- Bones—e.g., in a firm ball-and-socket joint such
as the hip joint, bony contours contribute to
stability.
- Ligaments—these act to prevent excessive
movement.
- Muscles.

In general, if a joint is very stable it has a reduced range of movement. For example, if you compare the stable hip joint with the less stable shoulder joint, the latter has a greater range of movement.

Muscle

There are three types of muscle in the human body.

- Striated skeletal muscle—voluntary somatic muscle that comprises the gross muscular system.
- Striated cardiac muscle—involuntary visceral muscle of the heart.
- Smooth muscle—unstriated, involuntary muscle in the walls of vessels and hollow organs (viscera).

Skeletal muscles and tendons

Skeletal muscles are aggregations of contractile fibers that move large structures, such as the skeleton, and organs, such as the eye, skin (facial muscle), and mucous membranes (tongue). They are joined to bone by tendons at their ends.

Skeletal muscle action

Muscles can be classified according to their action:

- Prime mover—the muscle is the major muscle responsible for a particular movement, e.g., brachialis is the prime mover in flexing the elbow.
- Antagonist—any muscle that opposes the action of the prime mover: it relaxes, but in a controlled manner, to assist the prime mover, e.g., triceps in flexion of the elbow.
- Fixator—prime mover and antagonist acting together to "fix" a joint, e.g., muscles holding the scapula steady when deltoid moves the humerus.
- Synergist—prevents unwanted movement in an intermediate joint, e.g., extensors of the carpus contract to fix the wrist joint, allowing the long flexors of the fingers to function effectively.

Skeletal muscle design

Muscle fibers may be either parallel or oblique to the line of pull of the whole muscle.

Parallel fibers allow maximal range of mobility. These muscles can be classified by shape:

- Quadrangular—four-sided, such as the pronator quadratus.
- Strap—or flat, such as the sternohyoid.
- Fusiform—spindle-shaped, such as the biceps brachii.

Oblique fibers increase the force generated at the expense of reduced mobility. These muscles are generally pennate or feather-shaped:

- Unipennate—such as the extensor digitorum longus.
- Bipennate—such as the dorsal interossei.
- Multipennate—such as the deltoid.

Circular fibers surround body openings, constricting them when contracted, such as the external anal sphincter.

Skeletal muscle organization and function

Somatic motor nerves control the contraction of skeletal muscle. Each motor neuron together with the muscle fibers it supplies constitutes a motor unit. The size of motor units varies considerably: where fine precise movements are required, a single neuron may supply only a few muscle fibers, e.g., the extrinsic eye muscles; conversely, in the large gluteus maximus muscle, a single neuron may supply several hundred muscle fibers. The smaller the size of the motor unit, the more precise the movements possible.

The force generated by a skeletal muscle is related to the cross-sectional area of its fibers. For a fixed volume of muscle, shorter fibers produce more force but less shortening.

Skeletal muscle attachments

Tendons are dense collagenous tissue that attach the ends of muscle to bone, cartilage, and ligaments by tendons. Some flat muscles are attached by a flattened tendon, an aponeurosis, or fascia.

When symmetrical muscle fibers unite at an angle (e.g., in the digastric muscle), a tendinous raphe is formed.

When tendons cross joints, they are often enclosed in a synovial sheath, a layer of connective tissue lined by a synovial membrane and lubricated by synovial fluid.

Bursae are sacs of connective tissue filled with synovial fluid, which lie between tendons and bony areas and bone and skin, acting as cushioning devices.

Cardiac muscle

Cardiac muscle is striated, like skeletal muscle, but with shorter, interdigitating fibers. It comprises the muscle of the heart (myocardium) and adjacent portions of the great vessels. Its action is involuntary, strong, continuous, and rhythmic, and it is innervated by the ANS.

Smooth muscle

Smooth muscle consists of small, nonstriated fibers found in the walls of blood vessels, hollow viscera, and the ciliary body of the eye, and comprises the arrector pili muscles. It is involuntary and innervated by the ANS.

Nerves

The nervous system is divided into the central nervous system (CNS) and the peripheral nervous system (PNS). The central nervous system is composed of the brain and spinal cord; the peripheral nervous system consists of the cranial and spinal nerves and their distribution. The nervous system may also be divided into the somatic and autonomic nervous systems. The sole target of somatic motor (efferent) fibers is skeletal muscle. Autonomic efferents innervate cardiac muscle, smooth muscle, and glands.

The conducting cells of the nervous system are termed neurons. A typical motor neuron consists of a cell body, which contains the nucleus and gives off a single axon and numerous dendrites (Fig. 1.9). The cell bodies of most neurons are located within the central nervous system, where they aggregate to form nuclei. Cell bodies in the peripheral nervous system aggregate in ganglia.

Axons are the nerve fibers, and they conduct action potentials generated in the cell body to influence other neurons or affect organs. Axons in the CNS and PNS can be nonmyelinated or myelinated, e.g., surrounded by a lipid-rich, insulating sheath interspersed with small gaps, called nodes of Ranvier, which allow for saltatory conduction of the nerve impulse.

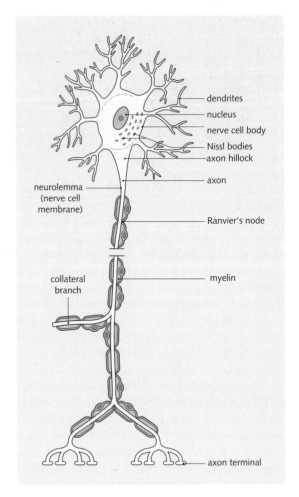

Fig. 1.9 Structure of a typical neuron.

Most nerves in the peripheral nervous system are bundles of motor, sensory, and autonomic axons. The region of the head is largely supplied by the 12 cranial nerves. The remainder of the trunk and the limbs are supplied by the segmental spinal nerves.

Autonomic nerves are either sympathetic or parasympathetic. In general, the sympathetic nervous system enables the body to deal with stress (so-called fight or flight responses). The parasympathetic system is primarily homeostatic, promoting the normal processes of the body such as peristalsis of the gastrointestinal system and the secretion of digestive juices.

Sympathetic preganglionic fibers arise from the thoracic and lumbar segments of the spinal cord. They synapse in a sympathetic chain ganglion, from which a postganglionic fiber can either enter a spinal nerve or innervate viscera. Some preganglionic fibers pass through the chain (splanchnic nerves) and synapse in prevertebral ganglia, e.g., celiac ganglion. The cell bodies of parasympathetic preganglionic fibers are found in the brain and sacral region of the spinal cord. These fibers synapse in ganglia associated with organs, e.g., a pulmonary ganglion, and postganglionic fibers from cell bodies in these ganglia innervate the organ.

Visceral sensory fibers, which carry poorly localized pain sensation from the viscera and are part of visceral reflex loops, travel centrally along either parasympathetic or sympathetic fiber tracts. They are not part of the autonomic system.

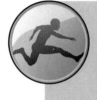

The importance of the myelin sheath to nerve conduction is well illustrated in multiple sclerosis, where focal loss of myelin leads to severe motor disability.

Spinal nerves

There are 31 pairs of spinal nerves: 8 cervical, 12 thoracic, 5 lumbar, 5 sacral, and the coccygeal nerve.

Each spinal nerve is formed by the union of the anterior and posterior roots (Fig. 1.10):

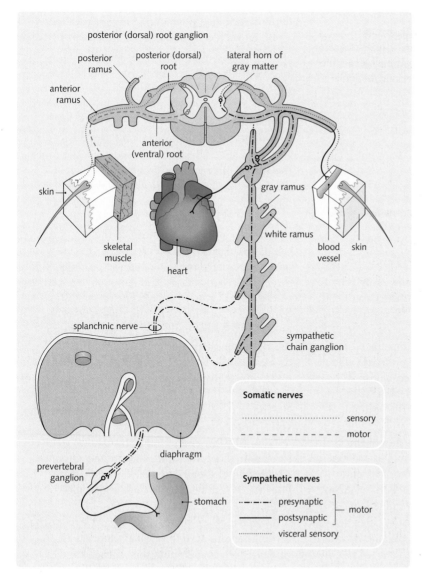

Fig. 1.10 Components of a typical spinal nerve.

- The anterior or ventral root contains motor fibers for skeletal muscles. Those from T1 to L2 also contain sympathetic fibers; S2 to S4 also contain parasympathetic fibers.
- The posterior or dorsal root contains sensory fibers whose cell bodies are in the posterior or dorsal root ganglion (DRG).

Immediately after formation, the spinal nerve divides into anterior and posterior rami. Both rami carry motor and sensory fibers as well as autonomics. The great nerve plexuses, e.g., the brachial, lumbar, and sacral, are formed by anterior rami.

Dermatomes

The area of skin innervated by the fibers of a single spinal nerve is called a dermatome. Dermatome maps have been drawn to indicate the normal pattern of skin innervation by specific spinal nerves. However, lesion of a single spinal nerve would rarely result in the loss of innervation to its dermatome because the innervation of adjacent dermatomes would overlap the affected one.

Circulatory system

The circulatory system consists of the cardiovascular and lymphatic systems and functions to transport fluids through the body.

Cardiovascular system

The cardiovascular system functions principally to transport oxygen and nutrients to the tissues and carbon dioxide and other metabolic waste products away from the tissues.

The right side of the heart pumps blood to the lungs via the pulmonary circulation. After returning to the heart, oxygenated blood is pumped by the left side of the heart through the aorta to the rest of the body via the systemic circulation.

Blood is distributed to the organs via thick-walled arteries to progressively smaller arteries, then to the smallest arteries (arterioles), and finally to capillaries. In a capillary bed, exchange of oxygen, nutrients, and waste products occurs, and then the blood passes into thin-walled venules, progressively larger veins, and finally back to the heart.

Valves occur principally in the veins of the limbs, where blood pressure is the lowest, to prevent back-flow of blood.

Metastasis of cancer cells is enabled by the free flow of blood through veins having no valves, such as the vertebral and pelvic veins and those of the head and neck.

Anastomosis

This is a communication between two vessels. Normally little flow of blood occurs through anastomoses; however, if an artery is occluded, the anastomoses assume greater importance in helping to maintain the circulation to structures distal to the blockage. If a vessel is slowly occluded, new vessels develop (collaterals) to provide potential detours for blood flow around an obstruction.

When such communications are absent between arteries, the vessel is known as an end artery. Occlusion in these vessels leads to necrosis, e.g., in the central artery of the retina.

Lymphatics

Knowledge of the anatomy of the lymphatic system is important to clinicians for predicting the route of the spread of cancer and infections. Fig. 1.11 illustrates the lymphatic system in the human body.

Most of the components of tissue fluid, in which cells are bathed, return to the cardiovascular system via capillaries. Excess fluid, including large plasma and cellular proteins, lipids, foreign microorganisms, and lymphocytes, returns to the venous system via lymphatic vessels as lymph. The lymphatics on the right side of the head, neck, upper limb, and thorax drain into the right lymphatic duct. The rest of the body drains into the thoracic duct. Both these ducts drain into the venous system near the right side of the heart.

Numerous lymph nodes located along the lymph vessels filter out cells, particulate matter, and microorganisms, and produce antibodies against foreign material, initiating an immune response. Absorption of dietary lipids from the small intestine is into lymphatic capillaries called lacteals.

Lymphatics are found in all tissues except the central nervous system, eyeball, internal ear, cartilage, bone, and epidermis of the skin.

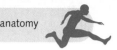

Fig. 1.11 The lymphatic system.

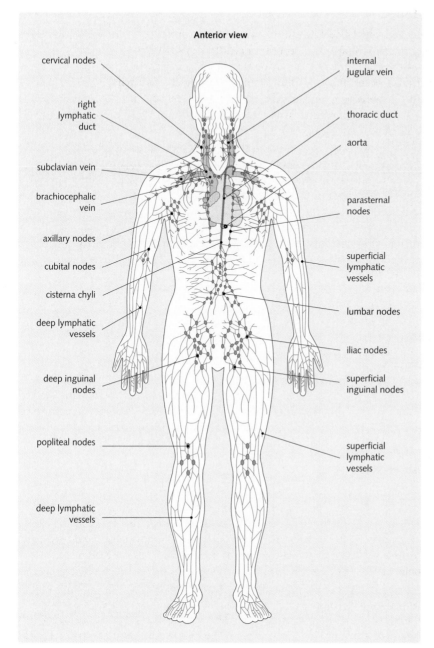

Anterior view

cervical nodes

right lymphatic duct

subclavian vein

brachiocephalic vein

axillary nodes

cubital nodes

cisterna chyli

deep lymphatic vessels

deep inguinal nodes

popliteal nodes

deep lymphatic vessels

internal jugular vein

thoracic duct

aorta

parasternal nodes

superficial lymphatic vessels

lumbar nodes

iliac nodes

superficial inguinal nodes

superficial lymphatic vessels

- Describe the anatomical position.
- What are the anatomic planes?
- Define the anatomical terms used in anatomy and clinical practice.
- Describe the terms of movement including the thumb.
- What are the appendages of the skin?
- What is the clinical significance of the compartments formed by deep fascia?
- Discuss the structure of a long bone.
- What factors contribute to the stability of the different kinds of joints?
- What are the classifications of skeletal muscles according to their action?
- Describe the differences in skeletal, cardiac, and smooth muscle in their structure, innervation, location, and function.
- Outline the components of a typical neuron.
- What is the function of the autonomic nervous system?
- What are the differences between the cardiovascular and lymphatic systems?

2. The Back

Regions and components of the back

The back consists of the vertebral column, the spinal cord, the roots of the spinal nerves, associated muscles, the posterior portions of the ribs in the thoracic region, and overlying skin and subcutaneous tissues.

The vertebral column extends from the skull to the coccyx. It is composed of 33 vertebrae arranged in five regions (seven cervical, twelve thoracic, five lumbar, five sacral, and four coccygeal). The sacral and coccygeal vertebrae fuse to form the sacrum and coccyx, respectively (see Fig. 2.2). The vertebral column thus supports the weight of the body above the pelvic girdle. Successive vertebrae increase in size as the column descends due to the increasing weight they bear.

Back pain is a nonspecific term for pain from a variety of sources. It is experienced by 80% of people during their lifetime and results from an upright stance and a bipedal gait. A few of the many factors that can cause back pain are dehydration and stiffening of the intervertebral disc with age, osteoporosis of the zygapophysial joints between the veretebrae, and weakened back and abdominal musculature, leading to poor posture.

There are four curvatures of the vertebral column in adults. The cervical and lumbar curvatures (secondary curvatures) are concave posteriorly; the thoracic and sacrococcygeal curvatures (primary curvatures) are concave anteriorly. The primary curvatures develop during the fetal period, whereas the secondary curvatures begin to develop when the infant begins to raise its head and hold it erect (cervical) and learns to stand and walk (lumbar).

Abnormal lateral curvature of the vertebral column, together with rotation of the vertebral spines toward the affected side, is called scoliosis. It can be caused by contralateral weakness in the intrinsic back muscles.

Surface anatomy and superficial structures

Visible and palpable features of the back are shown in Fig. 2.1. Note the following:
- The first easily palpable spine when passing a finger down the back of the neck is that of C7.
- The inferior angle of the scapula lies at the angle of the spine of T7 vertebra.
- A line passing through the highest point of the iliac crest passes through the spine of L4 verterbra.

The vertebral column

Skeleton of the vertebral column
The vertebral column consists of 33 vertebrae lying in five regions (Fig. 2.2). Individual vertebrae articulate with each other via intervertebral discs and articular facets (zygapophysial) joints.

The vertebral column supports the weight of the upper body. The weight is transferred to the lower limb via the pelvic girdle.

Although the movement between individual vertebrae is small because of the joints, ligaments, and muscles that connect them, the veretebral column overall is remarkably flexible and yet rigid to protect the spinal cord within it.

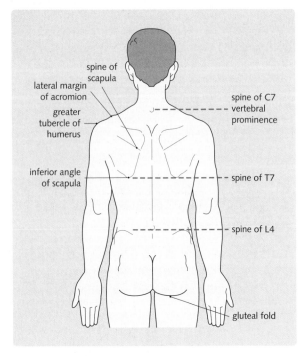

Fig. 2.1 Surface features of the back.

Features of individual vertebrae

A typical vertebra consists of:

- A body—the massive, cylindrical anterior part of the bone that supports the body weight; covered superiorly and inferiorly by hyaline cartilage to which the IV discs attach.
- A vertebral arch—consisting of pedicles, two short, cylindrical processes that project posteriorly from the body to meet the two flat plates of bone called laminae, which unite in the midline.
- A spinous process—projects posteriorly and inferiorly from the junction of the laminae.
- Two transverse processes—project posterolaterally from the junctions of the pedicles and laminae.
- Four articular processes—two superior and two inferior, which also arise from the junctions of the pedicles and laminae, each having an articular surface or facet.

See Fig. 2.3 for a typical vertebra, represented by L2.

Most vertebrae have characteristics that place them in one of the five regions of the vertebral

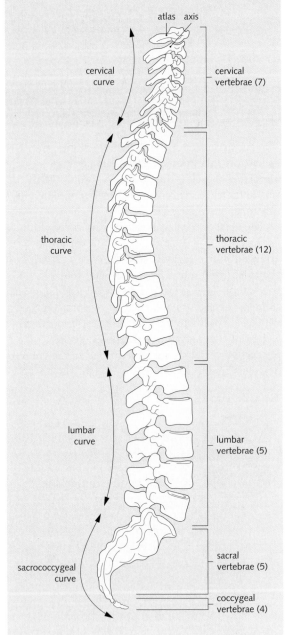

Fig. 2.2 Lateral view of the vertebral column.

column. See Fig. 2.4 for a summary of these regional characteristics and Figs. 2.3, 2.5, and 2.6.

The sacrum consists of five fused vertebrae (Fig. 2.7). The vertebral canal continues within the sacrum as the sacral canal. On the pelvic (anterior) and posterior surfaces of the sacrum are typically four pairs of sacral foramina for the exit of the

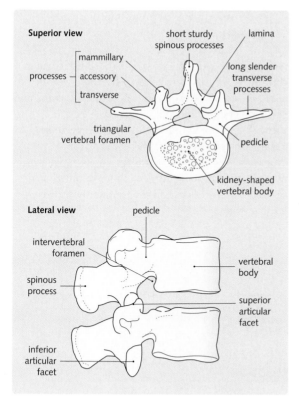

Fig. 2.3 Features of typical lumbar vertebrae.

posterior and anterior rami of the sacral spinal nerves. The anterior projecting edge of the body of SI is called the sacral promontory, a prominent obstetric landmark (see Chapter 7). On the dorsal surface, the median sacral crest represents the fused spinal processes of the sacral vertebrae. Intermediate sacral crests on either side of the midline represent the fused articular processes.

The sacrum articulates with the hip bone via its articular surface at the sacroiliac joint.

The coccyx or tail bone is small and triangular. It is formed from the fusion of four (three or five) rudimentary coccygeal vertebrae and fuses with the sacrum with age (see Fig. 2.7).

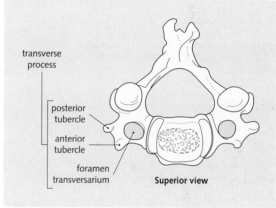

Fig. 2.5 Typical cervical vertebra.

Regional characteristics of vertebrae						
Region	Number	Body	Vertebral foramen	Orientation of facet joint	Spinous process	Transverse processes
Cervical	7	Small, wider from side to side	Large and triangular	Nearly horizontal	Short (C3–C5) Bifid (C3–C6) Long (C6, C7)	Have transverse foramina except for C7; transmit vertebral artery, vein, sympathetics
Thoracic	12	Heart-shaped, with 1–2 facets for articulation with the head of a rib	Circular, smaller than cervical and lumbar	Coronally oriented	Long, angled posteroinferiorly, overlap processes below	Long, extend posterolaterally, have facets for tubercle of rib
Lumbar	5	Massive and kidney-shaped	Triangular, larger than thoracic	Sagitally oriented	Short and thick; broad, hatchet-shaped	Long and slender

Fig. 2.4 Regional characteristics of vertebrae.

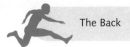

Intervertebral discs

Intervertebral discs are between and connected to adjacent vertebral bodies, and they are an integral part of the symphyses (secondary cartilaginous joints) between the bodies (Fig. 2.8). These joints provide strength and weight-bearing capacity, and they absorb compressive forces.

The disc is composed of:
- The anulus fibrosus—an outer ring made up of concentric layers of fibrocartilage.
- The nucleus pulposus—a gelatinous core that is more than 80% water, thus allowing the IV disc to act as a semi-fluid ball-bearing.

As people age, the nuclei pulposi lose their water content, becoming less turgid, and the layers of the anulus become thicker and can develop fissures and cavities. The nucleus pulposus may herniate through a degenerated anulus into the vertebral canal, compressing the spinal cord, or the intervertebral foramen, compressing the spinal nerve and its roots. This is commonly called a slipped disc and occurs most frequently in the lumbar region.

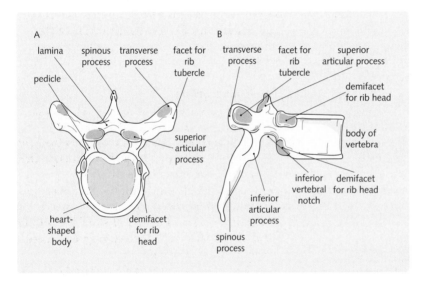

Fig. 2.6 (A) Superior and (B) lateral surfaces of a thoracic vertebra.

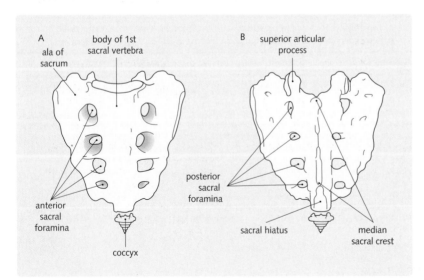

Fig. 2.7 (A) Anterior and (B) posterior views of the sacrum.

16

Herniation of the nucleus pulposus commonly occurs posterolaterally. Compression of the L5 and/or the S1 nerve roots causes lower back pain that radiates down the back of the lower limb.

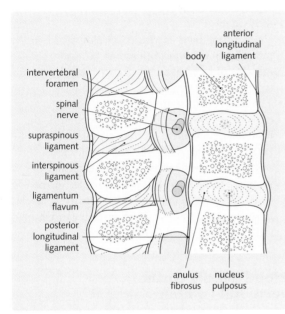

labels on figure:
- intervertebral foramen
- spinal nerve
- supraspinous ligament
- interspinous ligament
- ligamentum flavum
- posterior longitudinal ligament
- body
- anterior longitudinal ligament
- anulus fibrosus
- nucleus pulposus

Fig. 2.8 Sagittal selection of vertebrae showing the intervertebral discs and ligaments of the vertebral column.

Joints of the vertebral arches

These occur between the articular processes on the vertebral arches and are called facet (zygapophysial) joints. They are plane synovial joints, and their orientation affects the movements that can take place at the different vertebral levels.

Movement of the vertebral columns

The vertebral column is capable of flexion, extension, lateral flexion, and rotation. Mobility results from the compression and elasticity of the intervertebral discs (Fig. 2.9).

Atlanto-occipital joint

The atlanto-occipital joint is the articulation between the lateral masses of C1 vertebrae and the occipital condyles. It is a synovial joint surrounded by a loose capsule. Flexion and extension of the head occur at this joint ("yes-yes joint"), but no rotation.

Atlanto-axial joints

There are two lateral synovial joints between the lateral masses of the axis and atlas (Fig. 2.10). There is also a median pivot joint between the dens (odontoid process) of the axis and the anterior arch of the atlas. These joints allow rotational movement of the head in which the skull and the atlas rotate as a unit on the axis ("no-no joint"). Alar ligaments extend from the sides of the dens to the lateral margins of the foramen magnum; these prevent excessive rotation.

The transverse ligament of the atlas, which extends between the lateral masses of the atlas,

Movements of the vertebral column		
Vertebral region	Movements and accommodating factors	Limited movements and factors
Cervical	Flexion, extension, and lateral flexion occur because the intervertebral discs are thick compared with the vertebral bodies, facet joint capsules are loose, and the facet joints of C3 to C7 are sagitally oriented	Lateral rotation is limited due to the plane of the facet joints at C3 to C7
Thoracic	Rotation in combination with cervical rotation can occur because the plane of the facet joints lies in an arc, centered on the vertebral body	Flexion and extension are inhibited by facet joint shape, long spinous processes, the ribs, sternum, and thin intervertebral discs
Lumbar	Flexion, extension, and lateral flexion occur because of the large intervertebral discs and the sagitally oriented facet joints	Rotation is prevented by the interlocking articular processes of the facet joints

Fig. 2.9 Movements of the vertebral column.

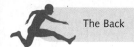

holds the dens against the anterior arch of the
atlas. Rupture of this ligament (e.g., during head
trauma) allows the dens to impinge on the cervical
spinal cord, causing paralysis of the body below
the neck. If the dens compresses the medulla, the
patient may die.

Ligaments of the vertebral column
These are shown in Fig. 2.8 and described in
Fig. 2.11.

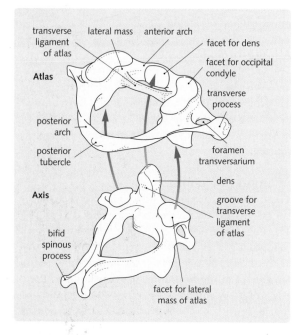

Fig. 2.10 Atlas and axis (showing their articulations).

Muscles of the vertebral column
An individual's body weight, for the greater part, is
anterior to the vertebral column. To support this
weight and move the vertebral column, there is a
strong mass of muscle that runs longitudinally on
the posterior aspect of the vertebrae, on either side
of the spinous processes. There are three main
groups of back muscles:

- The superficial extrinsic muscles connecting the
  upper limb to the trunk and producing limb
  movement—trapezius, latissimus dorsi, levator
  scapulae, and rhomboideus minor and major
  (see Chapter 3).
- The intermediate extrinsic muscles, which are
  more likely proprioceptive than accessory
  muscles of respiration—serratus posterior,
  superior, and inferior.
- The deep intrinsic muscles of the back,
  extending from the pelvis to the cranium and
  producing movement of the vertebral column
  (Figs. 2.12 and 2.13)—the superficial, thick
  splenius muscles, covering the underlying
  vertical muscles on the back and sides of the
  neck; the intermediate, vertical erector spinae
  muscle group; and the deep, obliquely oriented
  transversospinalis muscle group.

Blood supply to the vertebral column
Spinal arteries supplying the vertebral column are
branches of:

Ligaments of the vertebral column	
Ligament	Action
Anterior longitudinal	Strong band covering and connecting the anterior part of the vertebral bodies and the intervertebral disc. It runs from the anterior tubercle of the C1 vertebra to the sacrum; maintains stability of the joints between the vertebral bodies; and limits extension of the vertebral column
Posterior longitudinal	A narrow, rather weak band attached to the posterior aspect of the intervertebral discs and posterior edges of the vertebral bodies from C2 vertebra to the sacrum; weakly resists flexion of the vertebral column and posterior protrusion of the discs
Supraspinatus	A strong, cordlike band uniting the tips of the spinous processes; helps resist flexion
Interspinous	Weak, membranous sheets uniting the spinous processes; helps resist flexion
Ligamenta flava	Broad, yellow elastic bands uniting the laminae of adjacent vertebrae; helps to preserve the curvature of the vertebral column and support the joints between the vertebral arches

Fig. 2.11 Ligaments of the vertebral column.

Intrinsic muscles of the back			
Muscle	**Origin**	**Insertion**	**Action**
A. Deep intrinsic muscles of the back			
Deep layer			
Interspinales	Cervical and lumbar spinous processes	Spinous process of vertebrae above	Extension and rotation of vertebral column
Intertransversaii	Transverse process of cervical and lumbar vertebrae	Transverse processes of adjacent cervical and lumbar vertebrae	Lateral flexion and stabilization of vertebral column
Levatores costarum	Transverse processes of C7 and T1–T11	Transverse processes of adjacent vertebrae	Elevate ribs, assist in lateral flexion of vertebral column
Transversospinalis (intermediate layer)			
Rotatores	Transverse process	Lamina and transverse of 1–2 vertebrae above	Stabilization of vertebrae
Multifidus	Posterior sacrum and posterior superior iliac spine, transverse processes of T1–T3, articular processes of C1–C7	2–4 spinous processes above over entire length of spinous processes	Stabilization of vertebrae
Semispinalis	Transverse processes of C4–T12	Spinous processes above 4–6 vertebrea and occipital bone	Rotation of vertebral column and extension of head, cervical and thoracic regions
Erector spinae (superficial layer)			
Iliocostalis	All three originate from broad tendons from posterior sacrum and iliac	Angles of lower ribs, cervical and thoracic transverse processes, mastoid process,	As a muscle group, extension of vertebral column and head, control flexion by gradual lengthening of fibers
Longissimus	Crest, sacral and lumbar spinous processes	Same as iliocostalis	Lateral flexion when each is acting unilaterally
Spinalis		Spinous processes of upper thoracic vertebrae; cranium	
B. Superficial intrinsic muscles of the back			
Splenius capitis	Both originate from nuchal ligament and spinous processes of C7–T3 or T4	Mastoid process of temporal bone and superior nuchal line	Acting alone: lateral flexion and rotation of head
Splenius cervicis		Tubercle of transverse processes of of C1–C3 or C4	Acting together: extension of head and neck

Fig. 2.12 Intrinsic muscles of the back.

- Vertebral and ascending cervical arteries of the neck.
- Posterior intercostal arteries in the thoracic region.
- Subcostal and lumbar arteries in the abdomen.
- Iliolumbar and medial and lateral sacral arteries in the sacrum.

Periosteal branches of these arteries supply the vertebrae. Spinal artery branches enter the intervertebral foramina, supplying bone, periosteum, and meninges, and divide into radicular arteries. These supply the anterior and posterior roots of the spinal nerves and the spinal cord.

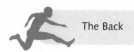

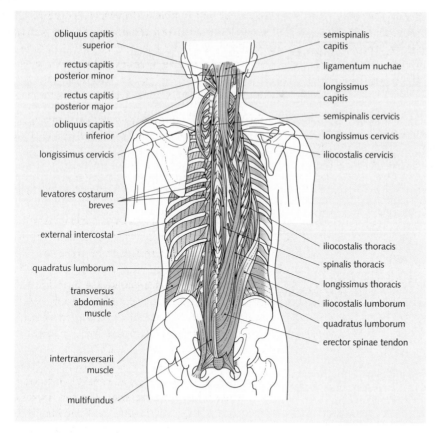

Fig. 2.13 Deep intrinsic muscles of the back. The right side shows the erector spinae components. Note that the longissimus cervicis has been moved laterally and the semispinalis capitis has been removed. (Adapted from Gray's Anatomy, 38th edn., edited by L. H. Bannister et al. Courtesy of Harcourt Brace and Co.)

Spinal veins form plexuses inside (internal vertebral venous plexus) and outside (external vertebral venous plexus) the vertebral canal (Fig. 2.14). Both plexuses have no valves and communicate with each other through the intervertebral foramina.

Blood may return from the pelvis and abdomen to the heart via the vertebral venous plexuses to posterior intercostal veins and from there to the superior vena cava. Abdominal and pelvic tumors may metastasize to the lungs in this way.

An aortic aneurysm or a cross-clamping of the aorta during surgery may lead to circulatory impairment of a segmental spinal artery and the compromise of the spinal cord segment supplied by this artery. This results in loss of sensation and voluntary movement below this level.

The suboccipital nerve has no cutaneous component.

Posterior neck

At the back of the neck are muscles that connect the skull to the spine and pectoral girdle. These are separated in the midline by a ligament, the ligamentum nuchae. The posterior neck is covered by the trapezius muscle superficially, and beneath the trapezius lie the splenius capitis and the splenius cervicis. These two thick, flat muscles cover and hold the deep muscles in position. Acting together or singly, the splenius muscles flex, rotate, or extend the head (see Fig. 2.12).

Ligamentum nuchae

The ligamentum nuchae is a strong, broad, fibroelastic ligament attaching superiorly to the

20

external occipital protuberance and inferiorly to the cervical vertebrae spinous processes. It provides muscular attachments for the trapezius and rhomboideus minor because the C3 to C5 spines are shorter than the other cervical spines.

Suboccipital region

This region is inferior to the occipital bone of the cranial base. Within this region is the suboccipital triangle, which is traversed by the vertebral artery before it enters the skull through the foramen magnum. The suboccipital nerve (C1) emerges from the triangle to innervate the muscles of this region.

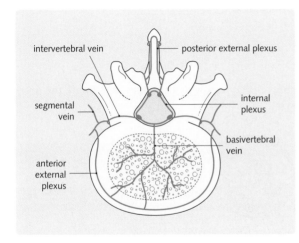

Fig. 2.14 Venous plexuses of the vertebral canal.

Four muscles are within this region (Fig. 2.15), three of which form the boundaries of the suboccipital triangle (Fig. 2.16):

- Rectus capitis posterior major (superomedially).
- Obliquus capitis superior (superolaterally).
- Obliquus capitis inferior (inferolaterally).

The fourth muscle, the rectus capitis posterior minor, lies medial to the triangle.

The spinal cord and meninges

The spinal cord lies in the vertebral canal. It is a continuation of the medulla oblongata that begins just below the foramen magnum and ends as a tapering region called the conus medullaris at the level of the L2–L4 vertebra in adults (Fig. 2.17). In children the spinal cord can end as low as the L4 vertebra. The bundle of spinal nerve rootlets from the lumbosacral region of the cord and the conus medullaris is called the cauda equina.

A cervical enlargement extends from the C4 to T1 spinal cord segments. Ventral rami from these segments form the brachial plexus. A lumbosacral enlargement extends from the L2 to S3 spinal cord segments. Ventral rami from these form the lumbar and sacral plexuses.

Blood supply to the spinal cord

One anterior and two posterior spinal arteries arise within the cranial cavity from the vertebral arteries or the posterior inferior cerebellar artery. Anterior

Muscles of the suboccipital region			
Muscle (nerve supply)	Origin	Insertion	Action
Rectus capitis posterior minor (suboccipital nerve)	Posterior tubercle of the posterior arch of atlas (C1)	Medial inferior nuchal line	Extend and rotate head
Rectus capitis posterior major (suboccipital nerve)	Spinous process of axis (C2)	Lateral inferior nuchal line	Extend and rotate head
Obliquus capitis inferior (suboccipital nerve)	Spinous process of axis (C2)	Transverse process of atlas (C1)	Rotate atlas and hence head
Obliquus capitis superior (suboccipital nerve)	Transverse process of atlas (C1)	Occipital bone between the nuchal lines	Lateral flexion

Fig. 2.15 Muscles of the suboccipital region.

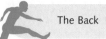

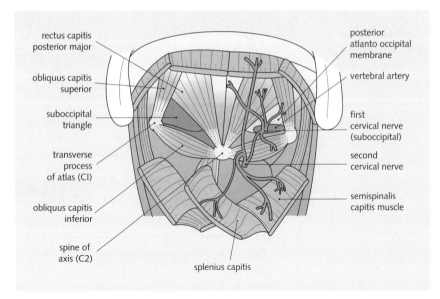

Fig. 2.16 The suboccipital region and contents. The right side shows the contents, and the left side shows the boundaries of the suboccipital triangle. (Adapted from Gray's Anatomy, 38th edn., edited by L. H. Bannister et al. Courtesy of Harcourt Brace and Co.)

Labels (left side, top to bottom): rectus capitis posterior major; obliquus capitis superior; suboccipital triangle; transverse process of atlas (CI); obliquus capitis inferior; spine of axis (C2); splenius capitis

Labels (right side, top to bottom): posterior atlanto occipital membrane; vertebral artery; first cervical nerve (suboccipital); second cervical nerve; semispinalis capitis muscle

and posterior radicular branches of the spinal arteries reinforce the blood supply.

Venous blood drains to the venous plexuses on the surface of the cord. These communicate with vertebral veins and dural sinuses in the cranium and with the internal and external vertebral plexuses.

Spinal nerves

There are 31 pairs of spinal nerves. Each is composed of a dorsal and ventral root (see Fig. 1.10). A level or segment of the spinal cord is specified by the intervertebral foramen through which the rootlets from or to that segment exit the vertebral canal (see Fig. 2.17).

Note that spinal nerves C1–C7 exit from the vertebral canal through the foramina above their respective vertebrae. From spinal nerve C8 and below all nerves exit through foramina below their respective vertebrae (see Fig. 2.17).

Cutaneous innervation of the back

The skin and muscles of the back are supplied segmentally by the posterior rami of the 31 pairs of spinal nerves. All posterior rami of the spinal nerves, except the first cervical nerve, divide into a medial and lateral branch. The posterior ramus of the first (suboccipital) cervical nerve supplies the deep muscles of the back of the neck (in the

suboccipital region), and it does not supply the skin.

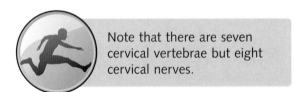

Note that there are seven cervical vertebrae but eight cervical nerves.

Spinal meninges and cerebrospinal fluid

The membranes called meninges and the cerebrospinal fluid (CSF) surround and protect the spinal cord.

Dura mater

The dura mater is a tough fibrous membrane forming a long, tubular sheath within the vertebral canal. It adheres to the margin of the foramen magnum, where it is continuous with the dura of the brain, and is anchored inferiorly to the coccyx by the filum terminale. It is separated from the vertebral periosteum by the epidural space. The dura mater extends into and adheres to the periosteum of the intervertebral foramina. It continues along the spinal nerve roots, investing them and eventually blending with the epineurium of the spinal nerves.

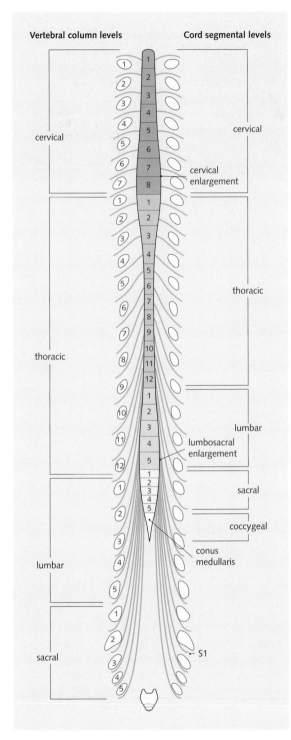

Vertebral column levels

Cord segmental levels

cervical

cervical

cervical enlargement

thoracic

thoracic

thoracic

lumbar

lumbosacral enlargement

lumbar

sacral

coccygeal

conus medullaris

lumbar

sacral

← S1

Fig. 2.17 Spinal cord, showing vertebral and segmental levels.

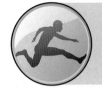

Remember that the adult spinal cord ends at the L2 vertebral level. The dural sac ends at the S2 level.

Arachnoid mater

The arachnoid mater is a delicate avascular membrane lining the dura mater and enclosing the subarachnoid space. A weak layer of cells is found between the dura and the arachnoid. Bleeding into this layer separates the arachnoid from the dura. This is called a subdural hematoma. Like the dura, the arachnoid mater covers the spinal nerve roots and spinal ganglia.

Pia mater

The pia mater is a finely vascular membrane that is closely adherent to the spinal cord. It covers the roots of the spinal nerve, the spinal ganglia, and the spinal blood vessels. Below the conus medullaris the pia continues as the pial filum terminale, which becomes invested with the dura of the dural filum terminale at S2 and attaches with the dura to the coccyx. The spinal cord is suspended within the dural sac by extensions of the pia called denticulate ligaments, which attach to the dural sac on either side.

Subarachnoid space

The subarachnoid space lies between the arachnoid and the pia mater. It thus surrounds the spinal cord, nerve roots, and ganglia. It contains CSF, which bathes and nourishes the spinal cord. An enlargement of this space inferior to the conus medullaris is called the lumbar cistern. It contains the cauda equina and extends from the L2 vertebra to the S2 vertebra.

Lumbar puncture

The spinal cord ceases at the level of the L2 vertebra, but the meninges continue well below this. By inserting a needle into the subarachnoid space below L2 in the region of the lumbar cistern, a sample of CSF may be extracted for analysis without damaging the cord.

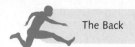

- Describe the components of the vertebral column and its curvatures.
- Describe the cutaneous innervation of the back.
- Describe the joints of the vertebral column.
- What is an intervertebral disc and its function?
- Describe the ligaments of the vertebral column.
- Describe the movements of the vertebral column.
- Describe the blood supply to the vertebral column and the spinal cord.
- Outline the boundaries and contents of the suboccipital triangle.
- Outline the spinal cord and its surrounding meninges.

3. The Upper Limb

Regions and components of the upper limb

The upper limbs are joined to the trunk by the shoulder or pectoral girdle. The shoulder region is the area around the shoulder joint and overlaps the superior aspect of the back and thorax and lower lateral neck. The arm connects the shoulder and the elbow. The forearm connects the elbow and the wrist. The hand is distal to the forearm and includes the wrist.

The pectoral girdle is a bony ring composed of the scapulae and clavicles. It is incomplete posteriorly but is completed anteriorly by the manubrium of the sternum. The scapula and clavicle articulate at the acromioclavicular joint. The sternoclavicular joint is the only joint between the shoulder girdle and the axial skeleton, and connects them together. All the remaining attachments to the axial skeleton are muscular. The humerus is the long bone of the arm, and it articulates with the scapula and with the ulna and radius. The radius and ulna articulate with the carpal bones of the hand at the wrist.

The subclavian artery is the major arterial supply of the upper limb. It arises from the brachiocephalic trunk on the right side and directly from the aorta on the left side. It continues as the axillary artery in the axilla and then in the arm as the brachial artery, which divides into the radial and ulnar arteries in the forearm to supply the forearm and hand.

Blood is returned to the axillary vein, which becomes the subclavian vein. Superficial veins drain into the axillary vein.

The nerve supply to the upper limb is derived from the brachial plexus: the median, musculocutaneous, and ulnar nerves supply the anterior compartments; the posterior compartments are supplied by the radial nerve.

Surface anatomy and superficial structures

Surface anatomy
Surface anatomy of the shoulder region is shown in Fig. 3.1.

Scapula
The scapula overlies the second through seventh ribs on the posterolateral thorax. Its inferior angle can be palpated opposite the T7 vertebral spine.

The spine of the scapula can be palpated subcutaneously from the T4 vertebral level medially to its lateral expansion as the acromion at the shoulder. The tip of the anterolaterally projecting coracoid process can be palpated deep in the deltopectoral triangle, a triangular hollow below the lateral third of the clavicle and bounded by the pectoralis major and deltoid muscles. The deltoid muscle forms the smooth rounded curve of the shoulder.

Axilla and axillary folds
The anterior and posterior axillary folds are skin and muscle tissue of the pectoralis major, and the teres minor and latissimus dorsi, respectively. The head of the humerus can be palpated only through the floor of the axilla.

Elbow region
The medial and lateral epicondyles of the humerus are subcutaneous on the medial and lateral sides of the elbow. The olecranon process, to which the triceps brachii tendon attaches, is separated from the skin only by the olecranon bursa; thus the overlying skin moves easily. The head of the radius can be palpated in a depression on the posterior aspect of the extended elbow, distal to the lateral epicondyle. The cubital fossa is a triangular hollow on the anterior surface of the elbow. The biceps brachii tendon is palpable as it enters the fossa, when the forearm is flexed against resistance.

Pulsations of the brachial artery may be felt deep to the medial border of the biceps bachii.

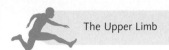
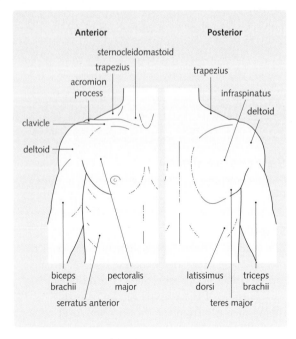

Fig. 3.1 Surface anatomy of the anterior and posterior views of the shoulder region.

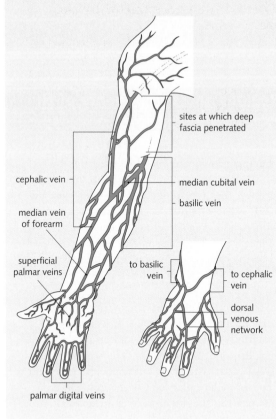

Fig. 3.2 Superficial venous drainage of the upper limb.

The radial styloid process is easily palpated on the lateral side of the wrist when the hand is supinated and abducted to the ulnar side. The head of the ulna is a rounded prominence at its distal end, which is easily palpated when the hand is supinated.

Superficial venous drainage

The dorsal venous network of the hand and the superficial palmar venous arch drain to the cephalic and basilic veins of the upper limb (Fig. 3.2), and they ascend in the forearm to the arm. The basilic vein ascends on the medial side of the forearm to about one-third of the way up the arm. It drains into the axillary vein. The cephalic vein ascends on the anterolateral aspect of the forearm, and it communicates with the basilic vein via the median cubital vein—this last vein is usually easy to identify because it passes obliquely across the cubital fossa, and it is frequently used for venipuncture. The cephalic vein continues laterally up the arm to the deltopectoral groove and then to the clavipectoral fossa, where it drains into the axillary vein.

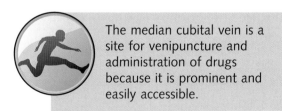

The median cubital vein is a site for venipuncture and administration of drugs because it is prominent and easily accessible.

Lymphatic drainage

Lymphatics in the hand coalesce to form trunks that ascend the forearm and the arm with the cephalic and basilic veins and the deep veins. Vessels accompanying the cephalic vein drain into the clavipectoral nodes or the apical axillary nodes. Some vessels along the basilic vein at the elbow, which enter cubital nodes, ultimately all drain into the axillary nodes. Deep lymphatic vessels, which drain the tissues, accompany major deep veins and terminate in the axillary nodes.

Cutaneous innervation of the upper limb

Figs. 3.3 and 3.4 illustrate the dermatomes and cutaneous innervation of the upper limb, respectively. This knowledge aids a differential diagnosis by indicating the level of a spinal nerve injury or lesion based on motor and sensory loss to a dermatome.

The shoulder region and axilla

Pectoral girdle

The pectoral girdle (clavicles and scapulae) and the bones of the upper limb form the appendicular skeleton (Fig. 3.5). The girdle itself is supported and provided with considerable mobility by muscles such as the trapezius, which attach to the

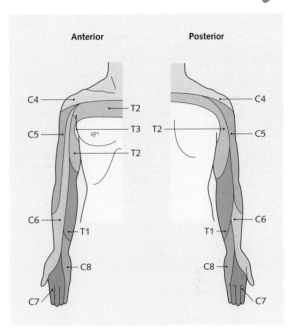

Fig. 3.3 Dermatomes of the upper limb.

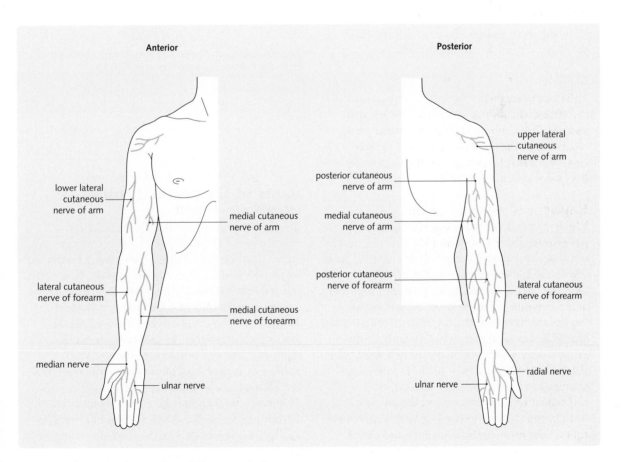

Fig. 3.4 Cutaneous innervation of the upper limb.

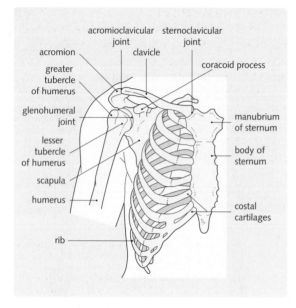

Fig. 3.5 Skeleton of the pectoral girdle.

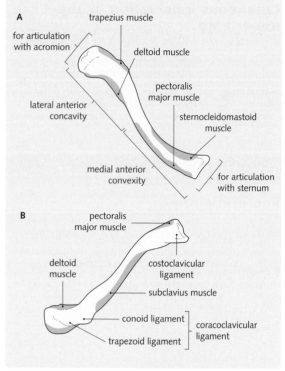

Fig. 3.6 Superior (A) and inferior (B) aspects of the right clavicle and its muscular attachments.

girdle as well as to the ribs, sternum, and vertebrae. It articulates directly with the axial skeleton only via the sternoclavicular joint.

Clavicle
The clavicle articulates with the sternum medially and with the acromion process of the scapula laterally (Fig. 3.6). Its shaft has a double curve in a horizontal plane. Fracture of the clavicle is common, and it usually occurs at the junction of the lateral and middle thirds.

Scapula
The scapula is a triangular flat bone lying on the posterolateral thoracic wall. It has superior, medial, and lateral borders, and superior and inferior angles (Fig. 3.7). The glenoid cavity, the main feature of the head of the scapula, articulates with the head of the humerus. A shallow constriction between the head and body of the scapula is termed the neck. The coracoid process is found above the genoid cavity and projects upward and anteriorly above the glenoid cavity; it provides attachment for muscles and ligaments.

The subscapular fossa lies on the anterior surface; the supraspinous and infraspinous fossae are on the posterior surface, above and below the spine of the scapula, respectively. The spine expands laterally as the acromion.

Joints of the pectoral girdle
Sternoclavicular joint
This is an atypical synovial joint because the articular surfaces are covered by fibrocartilage rather than hyaline cartilage. The joint is reinforced by the thickenings of its fibrous capsule, by anterior and posterior sternoclavicular ligaments, and by the interclavicular ligament superiorly. The joint is divided into two compartments by the articular disc, which is attached to the sternoclavicular ligaments. The costoclavicular ligament also stabilizes the joint by anchoring the inferior sternal end of the clavicle to the first rib.

As the lateral end of the clavicle is elevated, the clavicle can rotate around its longitudinal axis.

The joint is supplied by the medial supraclavicular nerve (C3–C4) from the cervical plexus and the nerve to the subclavius muscle.

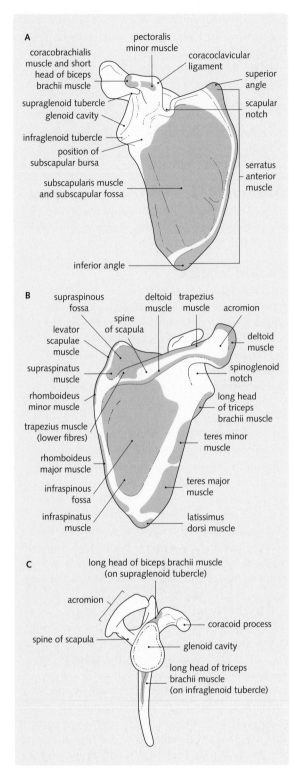

Fig. 3.7 Anterior (A), posterior (B), and lateral (C) aspects of the right scapula and its muscular attachments.

Acromioclavicular joint

This joint is found where the lateral end of the clavicle articulates with the medial border of the acromion. It is an atypical synovial joint, the articular surfaces being fibrocartilage.

A weak capsule surrounds the articular surfaces. It is reinforced by the acromioclavicular ligament superiorly and by fibers of the trapezius.

The coracoclavicular ligament is actually composed of two ligaments:

- The conoid, which attaches vertically to the inferior aspect of the clavicle.
- The trapezoid, which attaches more laterally and horizontally to the inferior clavicle.

This ligament is very strong and is a major factor in the stability of this joint.

The acromion of the scapula rotates on the acromial end of the clavicle. Since no muscles connect the bones at this joint, the movement of the scapula causes the acromion to move.

The joint is supplied by the lateral pectoral, axillary, and supraclavicular nerves.

Humerus

The upper end of the humerus is shown in Fig. 3.8. The head articulates with the glenoid cavity of the scapula. The surgical neck is the narrow part distal to the head and tubercles. The spiral groove of the humerus runs obliquely across its posterior surface for the passage of the radial nerve and the deep brachial artery.

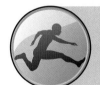

The surgical neck of the humerus is so called because it is a common site for fractures of the humerus.

Muscles of the upper limb

Fig. 3.9 outlines the major muscles of the upper limb.

Rotator cuff

The rotator cuff consists of the subscapularis, supraspinatus, infraspinatus, and teres minor. The tendons of these muscles surround the shoulder joint on all sides except inferiorly, and they blend with the joint capsule before inserting onto the humerus. They help to hold the large humeral head

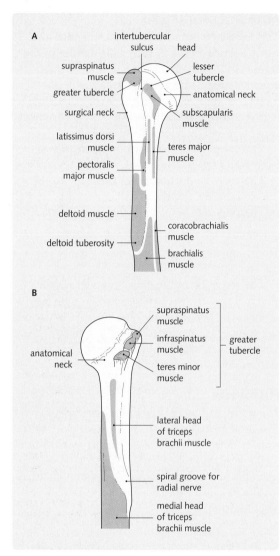

Fig. 3.8 (A) Anterior and (B) posterior views of the upper end of the humerus and its muscle attachments.

applied to the shallow glenoid cavity during arm movement.

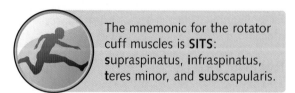

The mnemonic for the rotator cuff muscles is **SITS**: **s**upraspinatus, **i**nfraspinatus, **t**eres minor, and **s**ubscapularis.

Clavipectoral fascia

This is a strong sheet of connective tissue, deep to the pectoralis major, which attaches to the clavicle superiorly and splits to enclose the subcalvius and

pectoralis minor muscles inferiorly. It is continuous with the axillary fascia as the suspensory ligament of the axilla.

The following structures pierce the clavipectoral fascia:
- Cephalic vein.
- Thoracoacromial artery.
- Lymphatic vessels from the infraclavicular nodes.
- Lateral pectoral nerve.

Quadrangular and triangular spaces

Two notable spaces are formed by the arrangement of muscles and bones on the posterior shoulder (Fig. 3.10).

Shoulder joint

At the shoulder, or glenohumeral, joint there is articulation between the glenoid cavity of the scapula and the head of the humerus (Fig. 3.11). It is a multiaxial ball-and-socket synovial joint. A rim of fibrocartilage (called the glenoid labrum) is attached to the margins of the glenoid cavity.

The capsule surrounds the joint, which is attached to the margins of the glenoid cavity and to the humerus around the anatomic neck. A gap in the anterior part of the capsule allows communication between the synovial cavity and subscapular bursa, and an opening between the tubercles of the humerus allows for the passage of the long head of the biceps brachii. The capsule is strong but loose, allowing great mobility. It is strengthened by the tendons of the rotator cuff, except inferiorly, its weakest point. The synovial membrane lines the capsule, reflects back onto the articular margin of the head, and invests the long head of the biceps brachii in a tubular sleeve.

The glenohumeral ligaments are three thickenings. The capsule is reinforced superiorly by the strong coracohumeral ligament. The coracoacromial ligament spans the space between the acromion and the coracoid process and prevents superior dislocation of the humeral head.

The shoulder joint is inherently unstable owing to the very large head of the humerus compared with the shallow glenoid cavity. Factors stabilizing the shoulder joint are the glenoid labrum, all the ligaments, and the muscles supporting the joint. The nerve supply to the joint is from the lateral pectoral nerve, the suprascapular nerve, and the axillary nerve.

Major muscles of the upper limb			
Name of muscle (nerve supply)	**Origin**	**Insertion**	**Action**
Latissimus dorsi (thoracodorsal nerve)	Iliac crest, thoracolumar fascia, spinous processes of lower six thoracic vertebrae, inferior 3–4 ribs	Floor of intertubercular groove of humerus	Extends, abducts, and medially rotates humerus
Levator scapulae (C3 and C4 and dorsal scapular nerve)	Transverse processes of C1–C4	Medial border of scapula above root of spine	Elevates scapula and tilts glenoid cavity inferiorly by rotation
Rhomboideus minor (dorsal scapular nerve)	Ligamentum nuchae, spines of C7 and T1	Medial border of scapula at medial end of spine	Retracts scapula and rotates it to depress glenoid cavity
Rhomboideus major (dorsal scapular nerve)	Spinous processes of T2–T5	Medial border of scapula from spine to inferior angle	Retracts scapula and rotates it to depress glenoid cavity
Trapezius (spinal part of XI nerve [motor fibers] and C2 and C3 [sensory fibers])	Medial third of superior nuchal line, ligamentum nuchae, external occipital protuberance, spinous processes of C7–C17	Lateral third of clavicle, acromion, spine of scapula	Descending fibers elevate scapula, ascending fibers depress scapula, middle or all fibers retract scapula, descending and ascending fibers rotate glenoid cavity upward
Subclavius (nerve to subclavius)	Junction of first rib and its costal cartilage	Inferior surface, middle third of clavicle	Depresses and stabilizes the clavicle
Pectoralis major (medial and lateral pectoral nerves)	Medial half of clavicle, anterior surface of sternum, upper six costal cartilages	Lateral lip of inter-tubercular groove of humerus	Adducts arm, rotates it medially, clavicular head flexes humerus
Pectoralis minor (medial pectoral nerve)	Third, fourth, and fifth ribs near their costal cartilages	Coracoid process of scapula	Stabilizes scapula by pulling it anteriorly against thoracic wall
Serratus anterior (long thoracic nerve)	Lateral surfaces of upper 8 ribs	Medial border and inferior angle of scapula	Pulls scapula forward, holds it against thoracic wall, and rotates it
Deltoid (axillary nerve)	Lateral one-third of clavicle, acromion, spine of scapula	Lateral surface of humerus (deltoid tuberosity)	Anterior part: flexes and medially rotates; middle part: abducts; posterior part: extends and laterally rotates
Supraspinatus (supracapsular nerve)	Supraspinous fossa of scapula	Greater tubercle of humerus, capsule of shoulder joint	Initiates abduction of arm, helps hold humeral head in glenoid cavity
Subscapularis (upper and lower subscapular nerves)	Subscapular fossa	Lesser tubercle of humerus, capsule of shoulder joint	Medially rotates and adducts arm, helps hold humeral head in glenoid cavity
Teres major (lower subscapular nerve)	Posterior surface of inferior lateral border of scapula	Medial lip of intertubercular groove of humerus	Medially rotates and adducts arm
Teres minor (axillary nerve)	Lateral border of scapula	Greater tubercle of humerus, capsule of shoulder joint	Laterally rotates arm
Infraspinatus (suprascapular nerve)	Infraspinous fossa of scapula	Greater tubercle of humerus, capsule of shoulder joint	Laterally rotates arm

Fig. 3.9 Major muscles of the upper limb.

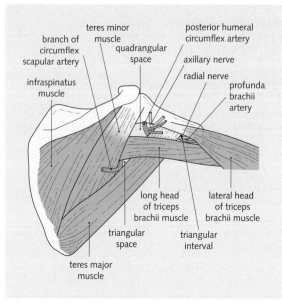

Fig. 3.10 Quadrangular and triangular spaces.

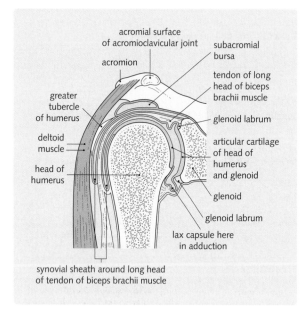

Fig. 3.11 Shoulder joint and related structures.

The movements at the shoulder joint, and the muscles performing them, are described in Fig. 3.12. The movement of abduction deserves special mention. The supraspinatus initiates the first 45 degrees of abduction, and the deltoid will abduct it to a maximum of 120 degrees at the glenohumeral joint. Further movement is obtained

by rotating the inferior angle of the scapula laterally and anteriorly, turning the glenoid cavity upwards. This is achieved by serratus anterior and trapezius.

The capsule of the shoulder joint is weak inferiorly and the rotator cuff is also deficient inferiorly. This is where dislocation of the humeral head can occur.

Axilla

The major vessels and nerves of the upper limb leave the neck to enter the apex of the axilla. The boundaries of the axilla are:

- Anterior wall: clavipectoral fascia, pectoralis major, and minor muscles.
- Posterior wall: subscapularis, latissimus dorsi, and teres major muscles.
- Medial wall: the upper four ribs, intercostal, and serratus anterior muscles.
- Lateral wall: intertubercular groove of humerus.
- The apex is the cervicoaxillary canal, which is bounded by the clavicle, first rib, and the superior border of the scapula.
- The base is composed of skin and axillary fascia, which extends from the arm to the thoracic wall and forms a hollow, the axillary fossa.

The contents of the axilla are shown in Fig. 3.13 and include:

- Axillary artery.
- Axillary vein.
- Brachial plexus.
- Axillary lymph nodes.

Axillary artery

The axillary artery is a continuation of the subclavian artery, and it commences at the lateral border of the first rib. Together with the brachial plexus, it is invested in fascia (axillary sheath), derived from the prevertebral fascia. The axillary artery becomes the brachial artery at the lower border of teres major. It is divided into three parts (Fig. 3.14):

Movements of the glenohumeral (shoulder) joint and the muscles performing them

Movement	Muscles
Flexion	Pectoralis major, anterior fibers of deltoid
Extension	Posterior fibers of deltoid, latissimus dorsi, teres major
Abduction	Deltoid, supraspinatus
Adduction	Sternocostal head of pectoralis major, latissimus dorsi, subscapularis, teres minor, infraspinatus
Lateral rotation	Infraspinatus, teres minor, posterior fibers of deltoid
Medial rotation	Pectoralis major, anterior fibers of deltoid, latissimus dorsi, subscapularis
Tensors of the anterior capsule (holding humeral head in glenoid cavity)	Subscapularis, supraspinatus, infraspinatus, teres minor
Resistance to downward dislocation of humeral head	Deltoid, long head of triceps, coracobrachialis, short head of biceps

Fig. 3.12 Movements of the shoulder joint and the muscles performing them.

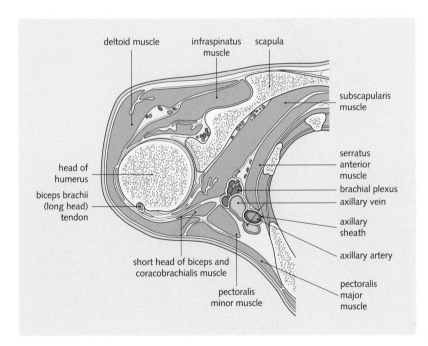

Fig. 3.13 Contents and muscular boundaries of the axilla.

- The first part lies betweeen the lateral border of the first rib and the medial border of the pectoralis minor and has one branch—the superior thoracic artery. This supplies the pectoralis major and the first and second intercostal spaces, and the thoracic wall.
- The second part lies posterior to the pectoralis minor and has two branches: (1) the thoracoacromial artery, which has four branches (the clavicular to the sternoclavicular joint, the pectoral to the pectoral muscles, the deltoid to the pectoralis minor and deltoid, and the acromial to the acromion), and (2) the lateral thoracic artery, which is the chief source of blood to the breast and also supplies the pectoral and serratus muscles.

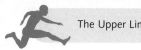

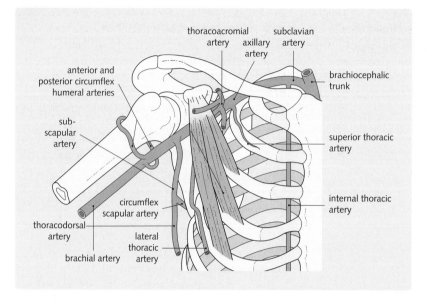

Fig. 3.14 Axillary artery and its branches.

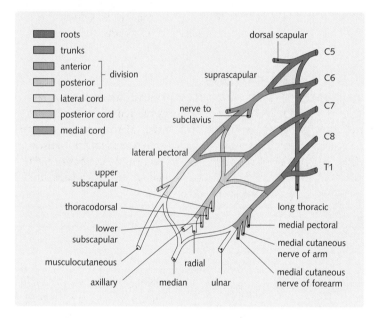

Fig. 3.15 Brachial plexus showing the trunks, divisions, cords, and branches.

• The third part passes from the lateral border of the pectoralis minor muscle to the inferior border of the teres major and has three branches. The first is the subscapular artery, which divides into two trunks: the circumflex scapular artery, forming part of a scapular anastomosis, and the thoracodorsal artery to the latissimus dorsi. The second and third are the anterior and posterior circumflex humeral arteries, which supply the shoulder joint and the deltoid muscle.

Axillary vein

The axillary vein is formed from the union of the brachial vein or veins with the basilic vein. It commences at the lower border of teres major and ascends through the axilla anteromedial to the axillary artery. At the lateral border of the first rib, it becomes the subclavian vein.

Brachial plexus

The brachial plexus is formed from the anterior rami of spinal nerve roots C5–C8 and T1. Fig. 3.15

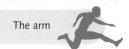

demonstrates that the plexus is divided into roots (deep to the scalene muscles); superior, middle, and inferior trunks (found in the posterior triangle of the neck); anterior and posterior divisions (behind the clavicle); and lateral, posterior, and medial cords (named with respect to their position around axillary artery). Fig. 3.16 tabulates the branches.

Notice, in Fig. 3.15, that the middle trunk of the brachial plexus as well as the lateral gives rise to an anterior division to form the lateral cord. All three trunks give rise to a posterior division to form the posterior cord.

Axillary lymph nodes
These comprise (Fig. 3.17):
- Lateral group medial to the axillary vein.
- Pectoral group along the inferior border of the pectoralis muscle.
- Subscapular group along the posterior axillary fold.
- Central group deep to the pectoralis minor, near the base of the axilla.
- Apical group at the apex of the axilla, on the medial side of the axillary vein. All the others drain to these nodes.

The arm

The arm lies between the shoulder and elbow joint. It has anterior and posterior compartments separated by the medial and lateral intermuscular septa. These septa arise from the deep fascia surrounding the arm.

Flexor compartment of the arm
The bony skeleton of the arm and the muscle attachments of the anterior compartment are shown in Fig. 3.18.

Muscles of the arm
The muscles of the arm are shown in Fig. 3.19. The coracobrachialis, biceps brachii, and brachialis

are found in the anterior, or flexor, compartment of the arm. The triceps brachii is the only muscle in the posterior, or extensor, compartment.

Vessels of the arm
Brachial artery
The brachial artery is a continuation of the axillary artery, commencing at the lower border of teres major (Fig. 3.20). It terminates in the cubital fossa at the neck of the radius under cover of the bicipital aponeurosis. There it divides into the radial and ulnar arteries. The brachial artery and its highest branch, the profunda brachii artery, supply the anterior and posterior compartments of the arm, respectively. Superior and inferior ulnar collateral branches of the brachial artery anastomose with recurrent radial and ulnar branches to form a collateral circulation around the elbow. The artery is relatively superficial throughout its course on the medial side of the humerus, behind the medial border of biceps brachii.

Brachial veins
Usually a pair of deep brachial veins accompany the brachial artery. They are joined by tributaries that correspond to branches of the brachial arteries and anastomose freely with the superficial veins and each other. The veins receive the basilic vein before becoming the axillary vein. Both superficial and deep veins have valves.

To remember the contents of the anterior arm compartment use the mnemonic **BBC** (**b**iceps brachii, **b**rachialis, and **c**oracobrachialis).

The brachial artery can be easily palpated on the medial aspect of the arm under biceps brachii.

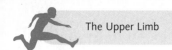

Branches of the brachial plexus and their distribution	
Branches	**Distribution**
Roots	
Dorsal scapular nerve (C5)	Rhomboid major, rhomboid minor, and levtor scapulae muscles
Long thoracic nerve (C5–C7)	Serratus anterior muscle
Upper trunk	
Suprascapular nerve (C5, C6)	Supraspinatus and infraspinatus muscles
Nerve to subclavius (C5, C6)	Subclavius muscle
Lateral cord	
Lateral pectoral nerve (C5–C7)	Pectoralis major muscle
Musculocutaneous nerve (C5–C7)	Coracobrachialis, biceps brachii, brachialis muscles, and the skin along the lateral border of the forearm (lateral cutaneous nerve of the forearm)
Lateral root of median nerve (C6, C7)	Joins the medial root (C8, T1) to form the median nerve (see below)
Posterior cord	
Upper subscapular nerve (C5–C6)	Superior portion of subscapularis muscle
Thoracodorsal nerve (C6–C8)	Latissmus dorsi muscle
Lower subscapular nerve (C5–C6)	Inferior portion of subscapularis and teres major muscles
Axillary nerve (C5–C6)	Deltoid and teres minor muscles, skin over the lower half of the deltoid muscle (upper lateral cutaneous nerve of arm)
Radial nerve (C5–C8, T1)	Triceps, anconeus, and posterior muscles of forearm, skin of the posterior and inferolateral aspects of the arm, posterior forearm, lateral half of the dorsum of hand, and dorsal surface of the lateral three and a half digits
Medial cord	
Medial pectoral nerve (C8, T1)	Pectoralis major and minor muscles
Medial cutaneous nerve of the arm (C8, T1)	Skin of the medial side of the arm
Medial cutaneous nerve of the forearm (C8, T1)	Skin of the medial side of the forearm
Ulnar nerve (C8, Ti)	Flexor carpi ulnaris and medial half of flexor digitorum profundus (in forearm) **Deep branch:** hypothenar, adductor pollicis, third and fourth lumbrical, interossei, and deep head of flexor pollicis brevis muscles (in hand) **Superficial branch:** palmaris brevis and skin of the medial half of the dorsum and palm of the hand, skin of the palmar and dorsal surfaces of the medial one and a half digits (palmar and dorsal digital cutaneous branches)
Median nerve (C5–C8, T1)	Pronator teres, flexor carpi radialis, flexor digitorum superficialis, lateral half of the flexor digitorum profundus, palmaris longus (median nerve in the forearm), flexor pollicis longus and pronator quadratus (anterior interosseus branch in forearm), thenar muscles (recurrent branch in each hand, first two lumbricals, skin of lateral half of palm and palmar surface of lateral three and a half digits (palmar and digital cutaneous branches)

Fig. 3.16 Branches of the brachial plexus and their distribution.

36

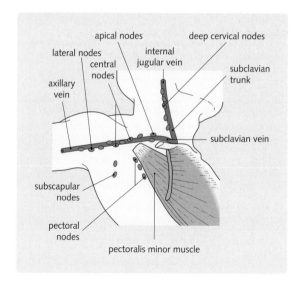

Fig. 3.17 Arrangement of axillary lymph nodes.

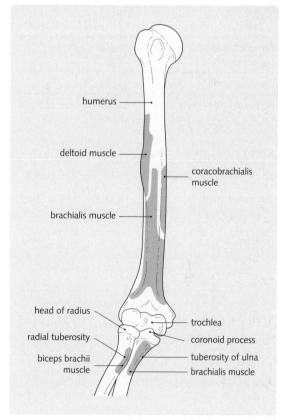

Fig. 3.18 Skeleton of the arm, showing sites of muscle attachment.

Nerves of the arm
Median nerve
The median nerve enters the arm on the lateral side of the brachial artery and in the middle crosses in front of the artery to be on its medial side. It continues to the cubital fossa in this relationship, and it is crossed by the bicipital aponeurosis. The median nerve has no branches in the axilla or arm.

Ulnar nerve
The ulnar nerve passes down the arm medial to the brachial artery and anterior to the long head of the triceps. It pierces the medial intermuscular septum halfway down, accompanied by the superior ulnar collateral artery, to enter the posterior compartment. It continues inferiorly between the medial intermuscular septum and the medial head of triceps, passing on the posterior aspect of the medial epicondyle of the humerus, and enters the forearm between the heads of flexor carpi ulnaris muscle. Pressure on the nerve as it crosses the medial epicondyle results in a tingling sensation— this area is referred to as the 'funny bone.' The ulnar nerve has no branches in the arm.

Radial nerve
The radial nerve enters the posterior compartment of the arm behind the brachial artery by passing below the lower border of teres major. It runs first anterior to the long head of the triceps and then inferolaterally with the profunda brachii artery, in the spiral groove of the humerus. The nerve pierces the lateral intermuscular septum to enter the anterior compartment of the arm and descends inferiorly between the brachialis and brachiordialis to the lateral epicondyle of the humerus.

Branches in the axilla and arm comprise muscular branches to the triceps and anconeus, and sensory branches to the posterior cutaneous nerve of the arm, the lower lateral cutaneous nerve of the arm, and the posterior cutaneous nerve of the forearm.

At the level of the elbow joint, the radial nerve provides muscular branches to brachioradialis and extensor carpi radialis longus.

Muscles of the upper arm			
Name of muscle (nerve supply)	Origin	Insertion	Action
Anterior fascial compartment			
Biceps brachii—long head (musculocutaneous nerve)	Supraglenoid tubercle of scapula	Tuberosity of radius and via bicipital aponeurosis into deep fascia of forearm	Supinates flexed forearm, flexes forearm, weakly flexes arm
Biceps brachii—short head (musculocutaneous nerve)	Tip of the coracoid process of scapula	Tuberosity of radius and via bicipital aponeurosis into deep fascia of forearm	Supinates flexed forearm, flexes forearm, weakly flexes arm
Coracobrachialis (musculocutaneous nerve)	Tip of the coracoid process of scapula	Middle third of medial surface of humerus	Flexes and abducts arm
Brachialis (musculocutaneous and radial nerve)	Distal half of anterior surface of humerus	Ulnar tuberosity and coronoid process	Flexes forearm
Posterior fascial compartment			
Triceps—long head (radial nerve)	Infraglenoid tubercle of scapula	Olecranon process of ulna	Extends forearm
Triceps—short head (radial nerve)	Posterior surface of humerus, superior to radial groove	Olecranon process of ulna	Extends forearm
Triceps—medial head (radial nerve)	Posterior surface of humerus, inferior to radial groove	Olecranon process of ulna	Extends forearm

Fig. 3.19 Muscles of the upper arm. (Adapted from Clinical Anatomy: An Illustrated Review with Questions and Explanations, 2nd edn., by R.S. Snell. Little Brown & Co.)

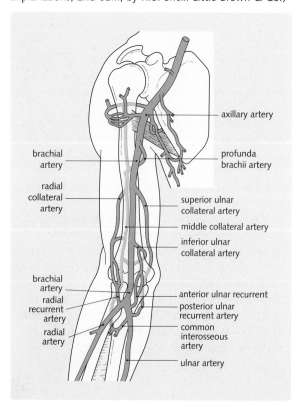

Fig. 3.20 Brachial artery and its branches.

The radial nerve runs in the spiral groove, and it can be damaged by midshaft fractures of the humerus. This paralyses extensor forearm muscles, causing wrist drop.

Musculocutaneous nerve

After its formation, the musculocutaneous nerve passes through coracobrachialis muscle and runs inferiorly between biceps and brachialis to reach the lateral aspect of brachialis. It supplies all three muscles of the anterior compartment, and it terminates by piercing the deep fascia lateral to the biceps to become the lateral cutaneous nerve of the forearm.

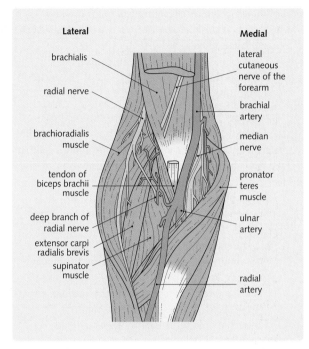

Fig. 3.21 Contents of the cubital fossa.

The cubital fossa and elbow joint

Cubital fossa

The cubital fossa is a triangular depression lying anterior to the elbow joint. Its boundaries are:
- Laterally—brachioradialis muscle.
- Medially—pronator teres.
- Superiorly—an imaginary line drawn between the two epicondyles of the humerus.
- Floor—the supinator and brachialis muscles.
- Roof—skin, brachial and antebrachial fascae, and the bicipital aponeurosis.

Fig. 3.21 shows the contents of the cubital fossa. Note:
- The radial nerve enters the anterior compartment between the brachioradialis and brachialis.
- The brachial artery crosses the tendon of biceps and the median nerve, deep to the bicipital aponeurosis.
- The proximal portions of the radial and ulnar ateries.
- The median nerve, medial to the brachial artery.

In the subcutaneous tissue over the fossa are the lateral and medial cutaneous nerves of the forearm, in relation to the basilic and cephalic veins.

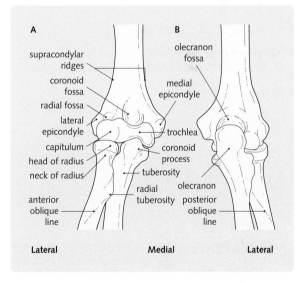

Fig. 3.22 Anterior (A) and posterior (B) aspects of the humerus and the upper end of the ulna and radius.

Elbow joint

The elbow joint is a synovial hinge joint between the lower end of the humerus and the upper end of the radius and the ulna (Fig. 3.22). Articular surfaces comprise:

39

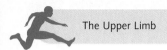
- The trochlea of the humerus medially and
- The capitulum of the humerus medially, which articulate with
- The trochlear notch of the ulna and
- The superior surface of the head of the radius, respectively.

Movements of the elbow joint are limited to flexion and extension. Independent rotation of the radius is possible at the proximal radioulnar joint in the movements of pronation and supination of the forearm.

The capsule is lax anteroposteriorly, but it is strengthened medially and laterally by collateral ligaments.

Ligaments comprise:

- The ulnar collateral ligament—this triangular ligament consists of three bands, and it extends from the lateral epicondyle of the humerus to the coronoid process and olecranon.
- The radial collateral ligament—this band extends from the lateral epicondyle of the humerus to the anular ligament.
- The anular ligament—this encircles and holds the head of the radius in the radial notch of the ulna, in the proxial radioulnar joint.

The nerve supply of the elbow joint and proximal radioulnar joint consists of:

- Musculocutaneous nerve.
- Median nerve.
- Ulnar nerve.
- Radial nerve.

 Remember that flexion and extension occur at the elbow joint; rotation occurs at the proximal radioulnar joint.

The forearm

The forearm lies between the elbow and wrist joints. It is roughly divided into anterior and posterior compartments by the radius, ulna, and the interosseous membrane (Fig. 3.23). The interosseous membrane is a thin strong membrane uniting the radius and ulnar bones at their interosseous borders. It provides attachments for some deep forearm muscles, and superiorly it is incomplete, allowing the posterior interosseus

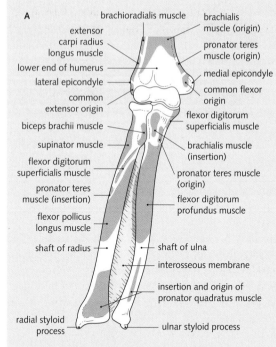

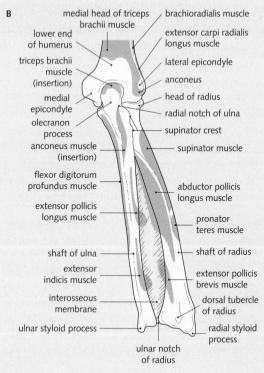

Fig. 3.23 Anterior (A) and posterior (B) aspects of the right radius and ulna, showing sites of muscular attachments.

vessels to pass, while inferiorly it is pierced by a small hole through which the anterior interosseous vessels pass to the back of the wrist.

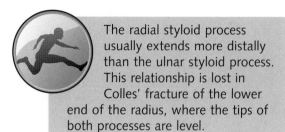

The radial styloid process usually extends more distally than the ulnar styloid process. This relationship is lost in Colles' fracture of the lower end of the radius, where the tips of both processes are level.

Anterior compartment of the forearm
Muscles of the anterior compartment
The muscles of the anterior compartment are flexors and pronators. They can be divided into superficial, intermediate, and deep groups (Fig. 3.24). The superficial muscles arise from the medial supracondylar ridge and the epicondyle of the humerus via a common flexor tendon.

Vessels of the anterior compartment
The brachial artery enters the forearm through the cubital fossa, where it divides into the radial and ulnar arteries (Fig. 3.25).

Just below its origin, the radial artery gives off a radial recurrent artery, which contributes to the arterial anastomosis around the elbow joint. The radial artery descends largely under cover of the brachioradialis muscle, together with the superficial branch of the radial nerve. It supplies the extensor muscles before emerging proximal to the wrist. Before turning laterally to reach the dorsum of the hand, it gives off a superficial palmar branch and a small palmar carpal branch to the wrist.

The ulnar artery gives off the common interosseus artery near its origin. This artery then divides into anterior and posterior interosseus arteries. The posterior interosseus artery enters the posterior compartment by passing above the upper border of the interosseus membrane, and it will be described in a later section. The anterior interosseus artery descends on the interosseus membrane, giving off muscular branches. It ends

in an anterior branch to the front of the wrist and a posterior branch that passes through a hole in the lower interosseus membrane to anastomose with the posterior interosseus artery and supply the dorsal wrist.

The ulnar atery itself gives off an ulnar recurrent branch that contributes to the anastomosis around the elbow joint, then descends through the forearm beneath the flexor carpi ulnaris to emerge at the wrist. At the wrist the ulnar artery gives off palmar and dorsal carpal branches to the carpal arches.

Nerves of the anterior compartment
The median and ulnar nerves pass through the anterior compartment. The median nerve is the principal nerve of the anterior compartment, innervating all of the muscles except the flexor carpi ulnaris and the medial half of the flexor digitorum profundus. The superficial branch of the radial nerve runs part of its course in this compartment.

Median nerve
This enters the forearm between the heads of pronator teres. It crosses the ulnar artery and then descends between the flexor digitorum superficialis and the flexor digitorum profundus. At the wrist, the median nerve is found deep to the palmaris longus tendon.

Branches of the median nerve in the forearm comprise:
- Anterior interosseous nerve. This leaves the median nerve in the distal part of the cubital fossa and passes through pronator teres. It joins the anterior interosseous artery and passes down the forearm on the anterior surface of the interosseous membrane between flexor pollicis longus and flexor digitorum profundus. It supplies flexor pollicis longus, the radial half of flexor digitorum profundus, and pronator quadratus, and it has articular branches to the distal radioulnar, wrist, and carpal joints.
- Muscular branches to the superficial and intermediate muscles except flexor carpi ulnaris.
- Palmar cutaneous nerve. This is given off just above the wrist joint. It supplies the skin over the central part of the palm of the hand.
- Articular branches to the elbow joint and proximal radioulnar joint.

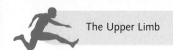

Muscles of the anterior compartment of the forearm			
Name of muscle (nerve supply)	**Origin**	**Insertion**	**Action**
Superficial			
Flexor carpi radialis (median nerve)	Common flexor tendon	Bases of second and third metacarpal bones	Flexion and abduction of wrist joint
Flexor carpi ulnaris— humeral head (ulnar nerve)	Common flexor tendon	Pisiform and through pisometacarpal ligament to fifth metacarpal bone	Flexion and adduction of wrist joint
Flexor carpi ulnaris– ulnar head (ulnar nerve)	Olceranon process and posterior border of ulna	Pisiform and through pisometacarpal ligament to fifth metacarpal bone	Flexion and adduction of wrist joint
Pronator teres— humeral head (median nerve)	Common flexor tendon and medial supracondylar ridge	Lateral aspect of shaft of radius	Pronation of forearm and flexion of elbow
Pronator teres— ulnar head (median nerve)	Coronoid process of ulna	Lateral aspect of shaft of radius	Pronation of forearm and flexion of elbow
Palmaris longus (median nerve)	Common flexor tendon	Palmar aponeurosis	Flexion of wrist joint
Intermediate			
Flexor digitorum superficialis— humeroulnar head (median nerve)	Common flexor tendon and coronoid process of ulna	Shafts of middle phalanges of medial four digits	Flexion of PIP and MCP joints of the medial four digits and wrist joint
Flexor digitorum superficialis—radial head (median nerve)	Superior half of anterior radius	Shafts of middle phalanges of medial four digits	Flexion of PIP and MCP joints of the medial four digits and wrist joint
Deep			
Pronator quadratus (anterior interosseus nerve)	Distal quarter of anterior surface of ulna	Distal quarter of anterior surface of ulna	Pronation of forearm
Flexor pollicis longus (anterior interosseus nerve)	Anterior surface of radius interosseus membrane	Base of distal phalanx of thumb	Flexion of interphalangeal MCP joints
Flexor digitorum profundus (medial half by ulnar nerve and lateral half by anterior interosseus nerve)	Proximal three quarters of anterior surface of ulna and interosseus membrane	Bases of distal phalanges of medial four digits	Flexion of DIP, PIP, MCP, and wrist joint

Fig. 3.24 Muscles of the anterior compartment of the forearm (DIP, distal interphalangeal; PIP, proximal interphalangeal; MCP, metacarpophalangeal).

Fig. 3.25 Arteries of the forearm.

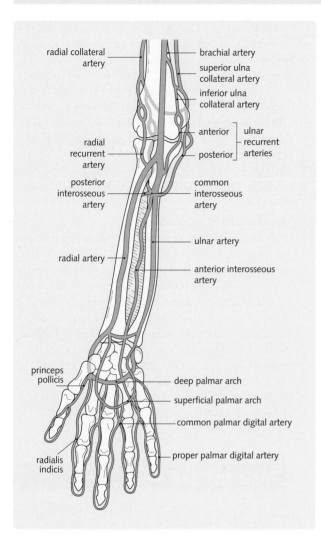

radial collateral artery

brachial artery

superior ulna collateral artery

inferior ulna collateral artery

radial recurrent artery

anterior

posterior } ulnar recurrent arteries

posterior interosseous artery

common interosseous artery

radial artery

ulnar artery

anterior interosseous artery

princeps pollicis

deep palmar arch

superficial palmar arch

common palmar digital artery

proper palmar digital artery

radialis indicis

The median nerve passes between the two heads of pronator teres to supply all of the muscles of the flexor compartment except flexor carpi ulnaris and the medial half of flexor digitorum profundus.

Ulnar nerve

This enters the anterior compartment by passing between the heads of flexor carpi ulnaris. It runs with the ulnar artery between flexor carpi ulnaris and flexor digitorum profundus. Proximal to the wrist, both artery and nerve become superficial on the lateral side of flexor carpi ulnaris.

Branches of the ulnar nerve in the forearm include:

- Muscular branches to flexor carpi ulnaris and the medial half of flexor digitorum profundus.
- A palmar cutaneous branch, which supplies the skin over the medial part of the palm.
- A dorsal branch, which passes deep to flexor carpi ulnaris to reach the dorsal aspect of the hand.

Radial nerve

This enters the forearm deep to the brachioradialis muscle. It divides in the cubtal fossa into a superficial and a deep branch. The deep branch passes laterally around the radius, piercing the supinator to enter the extensor compartment as the posterior interosseous nerve. The superficial branch continues down the forearm deep to brachioradialis, and it is joined by the radial artery. Both pass onto the dorsum of the hand.

Remember, the radial nerve supplies the posterior compartment of the arm, then pierces the supinator muscle to supply the extensor forearm muscles.

Posterior compartment of the forearm

Muscles of the posterior compartment

The superficial group of muscles arises from the lateral epicondyle (the common extensor origin) and the supracondylar ridge of the humerus. The deep group of muscles consists of a supinator of the forearm and muscles that extend the thumb and medial four digits (Figs. 3.23 and 3.26).

Vessels of the posterior compartment

The posterior interosseous artery from the ulnar artery passes posteriorly above the upper border of the interosseous membrane, accompanied by the posterior interosseous nerve. This artery supplies the deep and superficial muscles of the extensor compartment.

Nerves of the posterior compartment

The brachioradialis and extensor carpi radialis longus are supplied directly by the radial nerve. The supinator and extensor carpi radialis brevis are supplied by the deep branch of the radial nerve, while all the other extensor muscles are supplied by the posterior interosseous nerve from the deep branch.

This nerve emerges from supinator and runs on the interosseous membrane as far as the wrist joint, which it supplies.

Anatomic snuffbox

This is a depression proximal to the base of the first metacarpal and overlying the scaphoid and trapezoid bones that can be seen when the thumb is fully extended and abducted. The radial margin is formed by the tendons of abductor pollicis longus and extensor pollicis brevis.

The ulnar margin is formed by the tendon of extensor pollicis longus. The radial artery runs through the anatomic snuffbox on its course to the dorsum of the hand. It lies on the scaphoid bone here.

Acute tenderness in this region following a fall indicates a probable fracture of the scaphoid bone.

Radioulnar joints

The movements of pronation and supination occur at the proximal and distal radioulnar joints. In the proximal radioulnar joint, the head of the radius rotates in an osseofibrous ring formed by the radial notch of the ulna and the anular ligament. The head of the ulna articulates with the ulnar notch at the distal end of the radius in the distal radioulnar joint. A fibrocartilagenous articular disc binds the ends of the two bones within the joint, and the radius rotates around the ulna.

Biceps brachii and supinator cause supination, whereas pronator teres and quadratus are responsible for pronation.

The wrist and hand

Fig. 3.27 shows the skeleton of the wrist and hand.

Radiocarpal (wrist) joint

This is a synovial joint in which the distal end of the radius and the articular disc of the distal radioulnar joint articulate with the scaphoid, lunate, and triquetral bones (Fig. 3.28). The joint is strengthened by palmar radiocarpal and radioulnar and ulnar and radial collateral ligaments. The nerve supply to the joint is from anterior and posterior interosseous nerves.

Movements of the wrist joint are inseparable, functionally, from those at the intercarpal and midcarpal joint (synovial joints between the proximal and distal rows of carpal bones):
- Flexion.
- Extension.
- Radial abduction.
- Ulnar abduction (adduction).

Adduction is greater than abduction.

Muscles of the posterior compartment of the forearm			
Name of muscle (nerve supply)	Origin	Insertion	Action
Superficial			
Brachioradialis (radial nerve)	Lateral supracondylar ridge of humerus	Lateral surface of radius	Flexes forearm when it is in semi-prone position
Extensor carpi radialis longus (radial nerve)	Lateral supracondylar ridge of humerus	Dorsal base of second metacarpal bone	Extends and abducts hand at wrist joint
Extensor carpi radialis brevis (deep branch of radial nerve)	Common extensor tendon	Dorsal base of third metacarpal bone	Extends and abducts hand
Extensor digitorum (posterior interosseus nerve)	Common extensor tendon	Extensor expansion of middle and distal phalanges of the medial four digits	Extends the medial four fingers and hand at wrist joint
Extensor digiti minimi (postrerior interosseus nerve)	Common extensor tendon	Extensor expansion of little finger	Extends little finger
Extensor carpi ulnaris (posterior interosseus nerve)	Common extensor tendon	Base of fifth metacarpal bone	Extends and adducts hand at the wrist
Anconeus (radial nerve)	Commn extensor tendon	Olecranon process and shaft of ulna	Extends and stabilizes the elbow joint
Deep			
Supinator (deep branch of radial nerve)	Lateral epidondyle, supinator fossa, and crest of ulna	Neck and shaft of radius	Supinates forearm
Abductor pollicis longus (posterior interosseus nerve)	Posterior surface, proximal half of shafts of radius and ulna and interosseus membrane	Base of first metacarpal bone	Abducts thumb and extends at carpometacarpal joint
Extensor pollicis brevis (posterior interosseus nerve)	Posterior surface, distal third of shaft of radius and interosseus membrane	Base of proximal phalanx of thumb	Exends metacarpophalangeal joint of thumb
Extensor pollicis longus (posterior interosseus nerve)	Posterior third of shaft of ulna and interosseus membrane	Base of distal phalanx of thumb	Extends thumb
Extensor indicis (posterior interosseus nerve)	Posterior third of shaft of ulna and interosseus membrane	Extensor expansion of index finger	Extends index finger

Fig. 3.26 Muscles of the posterior compartment of the forearm.

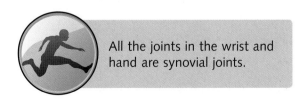

All the joints in the wrist and hand are synovial joints.

Dorsum of the hand

The skin on the dorsum of the hand is thin and loose, and a dorsal venous network of veins is usually visible. The veins drain into the cephalic and basilic veins.

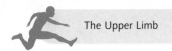

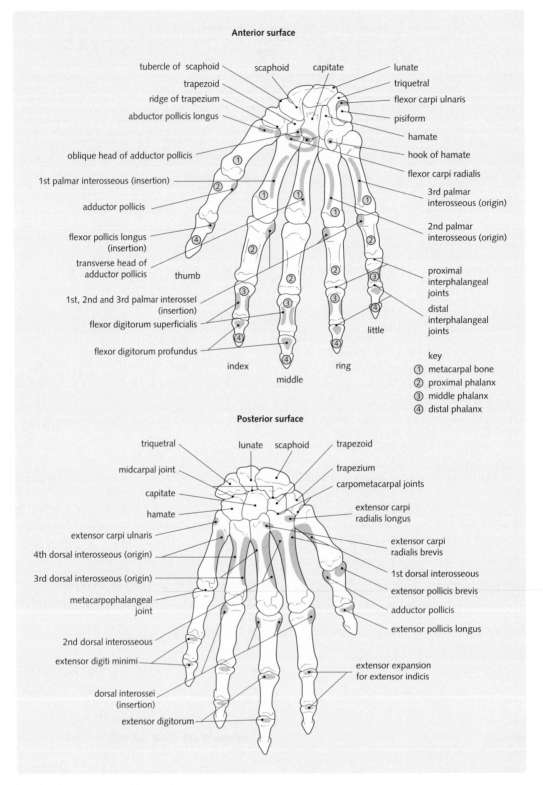

Fig. 3.27 Bones and joints of the wrist and hand.

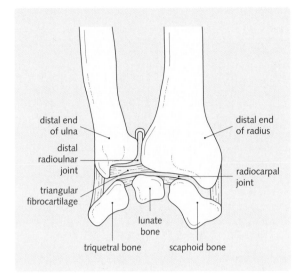

Fig. 3.28 Relationship of the distal radioulnar joint to the radiocarpal joint.

The long extensor tendons of the forearm lie beneath the superficial veins. As the tendons cross the wrist joint, they are surrounded by synovial sheaths and bound down by the extensor retinaculum to prevent bowstringing of the tendons when the hand is extended at the wrist. The extensor retinaculum attachments run from the radius to the pisiform and triquetral bones.

Six fibrotendinous tunnels, each lined with a synovial sheath, are formed by the slips of the extensor retinaculum to the radius and ulna and contain the twelve tendons of the nine extensor muscles.

Intertendinous connections join the four tendons of the extensor digitorum to one another, and they can be seen pulling on the tendons beneath the skin when the fingers are flexed.

The extensor tendons divide into three slips over the proximal phalanx: a central part that inserts into the middle phalanx, and two collateral bands that insert into the distal phalanx. These collateral bands receive a strong attachment from the interossei and lumbrical tendons. It is this attachment that forms the dorsal digital extensor expansion (Fig. 3.29).

The dorsal interossei are the only intrinsic muscles of the dorsum of the hand.

Nerve supply to the dorsum of the hand

Fig. 3.30 shows the cutaneous innervation of the hand. Note the fingertips are supplied by

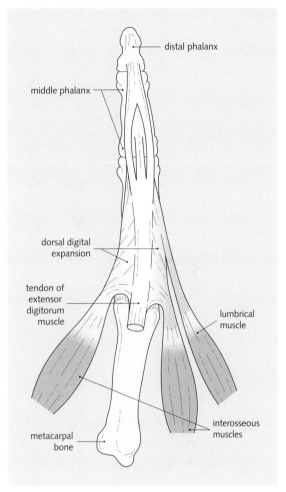

Fig. 3.29 Dorsal digital expansion and extensor tendon.

palmar digital branches of the median and ulnar nerves.

Vessels of the dorsum of the hand

Fig. 3.31 shows the blood supply to the dorsum of the hand.

Palm of the hand
Skin

The skin is thick and hairless. Flexure creases and papillary ridges occupy the entire flexor surface, improving the gripping ability of the hand. Fibrous bands bind the skin down to the palmar aponeurosis, dividing the subcutaneous fat into lobulated pads and preventing the skin from sliding when an object is gripped. A small palmaris brevis muscle attaches the dermis of the skin over the ulnar border of the hand to the palmar aponeurosis and flexor retinaculum. Its action of wrinkling the

47

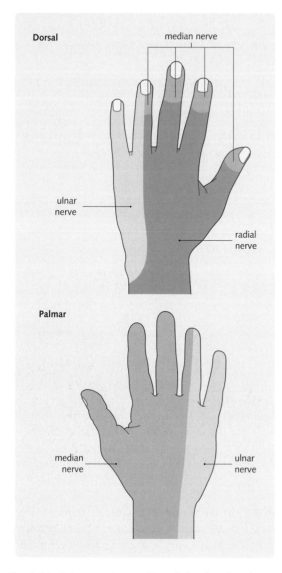

Fig. 3.30 Cutaneous innervation of the dorsal and palmar surfaces of the hand.

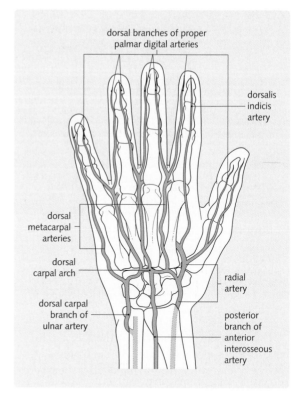

Fig. 3.31 Vessels of the dorsum of the hand.

skin over the hypothenar eminence and deepening the hollow of the palm improves the ability to grip objects.

Palmar aponeurosis
The palmar aponeurosis is a strong sheet of deep fascia lying between the thenar and hypothenar eminences, where it is continuous with the flexor retinaculum and the palmaris longus proximally. Distally it separates into four slips, which are attached to the base of each proximal phalanx and

become continuous with the fibrous flexor sheaths. Some fibers pass dorsally to attach to the metacarpals and the deep transverse metacarpal ligaments.

A shortening and thickening of the fibers of the palmar aponeurosis lead to fixed flexion of the digits (Dupuytren's contracture), which affects most severely the ring and little fingers.

Flexor retinaculum
The flexor retinaculum is a thickening of the antebrachial fascia in the front of the wrist that attaches distally to the scaphoid and trapezium on the lateral side and to the pisiform and hook of the hamate medially. This converts the concavity created by the carpal bones to an osseofibrous canal, called the carpal tunnel (Fig. 3.32). The flexor digitorum superficialis tendons enter the tunnel in two rows. The middle and ring finger tendons lie superficial to those of the index and little finger tendons. The flexor digitorum profundus tendons all lie in the same plane beneath the superficialis tendons. At the distal row of

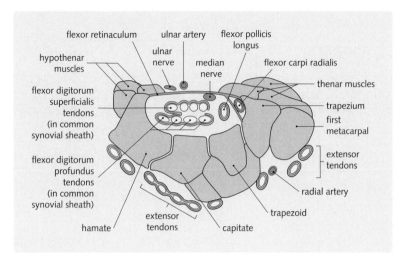

flexor retinaculum   ulnar artery   flexor pollicis longus

hypothenar muscles

ulnar nerve

median nerve

flexor carpi radialis

flexor digitorum superficialis tendons (in common synovial sheath)

thenar muscles

trapezium

first metacarpal

flexor digitorum profundus tendons (in common synovial sheath)

extensor tendons

radial artery

hamate

extensor tendons

trapezoid

capitate

Fig. 3.32 Cross-section of the right carpal tunnel at the distal row of carpal bones showing its contents. (Adapted from Gray's Anatomy, 38th edn., edited by L. H. Bannister et al. Harcourt Brace and Co.)

carpal bones the superficialis tendons all lie in the same plane. The remaining contents are the flexor pollicis longus tendon and median nerve on the radial side.

Compression of the median nerve in the carpal tunnel due to fluid retention, infection, or excessive exercise of the fingers results in weakening of the thenar muscles and anesthesia of the lateral three-and-a-half digits. This is known as carpal tunnel syndrome. Surgical division of the flexor retinaculum relieves the pressure and symptoms.

Muscles of the hand
Thenar eminence
The thenar eminence is the prominent region between the base of the thumb and the wrist. It is composed of three muscles (abductor pollicis brevis, flexor pollicis brevis, and opponens pollicis), the nerves and vessels to those muscles, and the overlying fat pad (Fig. 3.33).

Hypothenar eminence
The hypothenar eminence lies between the base of the small finger and the wrist. It consists of the abductor digiti minimi, flexor digiti minimi, and opponens digiti minimi; the nerves and vessels to those muscles; and the overlying fat pad (see Fig. 3.33).

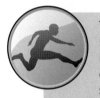

The recurrent branch of the median nerve supplies the muscles of the thenar eminence; the ulnar nerve supplies the muscles of the hypothenar eminence.

Other intrinsic hand muscles
These include adductor pollicis, lumbrical, palmaris brevis, and dorsal and palmar interosseous muscles (see Fig. 3.33).

The dorsal interossei (four) abduct the second, third, and fourth digits away from the cental axis of the hand, which is represented by the third (middle) finger. The palmar interossei (three) adduct the second, fourth, and fifth digits toward this axis. They, along with the lumbrical muscles, extend the interphalangeal joints and flex the metacarpophalangeal joints. This is due to the insertion of the interossei and lumbricals dorsal to the proximal phalanx, which causes flexion at the metacarpophalangeal joint. The interossei and lumbricals pull on their insertion into the extensor expansion, causing extension at the interphalangeal joints. This is a simple explanation to a rather complex action.

49

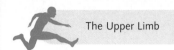

The intrinsic muscles of the hand			
Name of muscle (nerve supply)	Origin	Insertion	Action
Thenar muscles			
Abductor pollicis brevis (recurrent branch of median nerve)	Scaphoid, trapezium, and flexor retinaculum	Lateral side, base of proximal phalanx	Abducts thumb at the MCP joint
Flexor pollicis brevis (superficial head: recurrent branch of median nerve; deep head: deep branch of ulnar nerve)	Scaphoid, trapezium, and flexor retinaculum	Lateral side, base of proximal phalanx	Flexes thumb at the MCP joint
Opponens pollicis (recurrent branch of median nerve)	Scaphoid, trapezium, and flexor retinaculum	Lateral side, first metacarpal bone	Rotates metacarpal medially and draws it to the middle of of the palm
Adductor pollicis (deep branch of the ulnar nerve)	Oblique head: capitate, trapezoid, and second and third metacarpals; transverse head: anterior suface of third metacarpal	Medial side, base of proximal phalanx	Adducts thumb toward lateral border of palm
Hypothenar muscles			
Abductor digiti minimi (deep branch of ulnar nerve)	Pisiform and flexor retinaculum	Medial side, base of proximal phalanx	Abducts little finger at the MCP joint
Flexor digiti mimimi (deep branch of ulnar nerve)	Hook of hamate and flexor retinaculum	Medial side, base of proximal phalanx	Flexes proximal phalanx of the fifth digit at MCP joint
Opponens digiti minimi (deep branch of ulnar nerve)	Hook of hamate and flexor retinaculum	Medial side of fifth metacarpal bone	Draws fifth metacarpal centrally and rotates it to assist in gripping
Other intrinsic hand muscles			
Lumbricals (first and second: median nerve; third and fourth: deep branch of ulnar nerve)	Tendons of flexor digitorum profundus	Lateral (radial) sides of extensor expansion of the medial four digits	Extend the DIP and PIP joints of medial four digits and flex the MCP joints of medial four digits
Palmar interossei (deep branch of ulnar nerve)	Second, fourth, and fifth metacarpal bones	Base of the proximal phalanx and extensor of second to fifth digits	Adduct the digits toward the axis down the middle of the third digit, flex digits at MCP, and extend interphalangeal joints
Dorsal interossei (deep branch of ulnar nerve)	Adjacent sides of the five metacarpal bones	Base of proximal phalanx and extensor expanion of second to fourth digits	Abduct the digits away from the axis down the middle of the third digit, flex digits at MCP, and extend interphalangeal joints
Palmaris brevis (superficial branch of ulnar nerve)	Palmar aponeurosis of flexor retinaculum	Dermis of the skin on medial border of hand	Wrinkles the skin over the hypothenar eminence and deepens hollow of palm to improve the grip of the hand

Fig. 3.33 The intrinsic muscles of the hand.

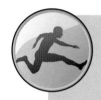

Use the mnemonics **DAB** and **PAD** to remember the actions of dorsal and palmar interossei: **DAB** = **d**orsal, **ab**duct and **PAD** = **p**almar, **ad**duct.

Long flexor tendons in the hand

The following flexor tendons enter the hand beneath the flexor retinaculum: flexor carpi radialis, flexor digitorum superficialis and profundus, and flexor pollicis longus.

The muscle tendons are surrounded by synovial sheaths as they pass beneath the retinaculum, and as they enter the digits.

Synovial flexor tendon sheaths

There is a common synovial sheath for flexor digitorum superficialis and profundus. The tendons of the flexor pollicis longus and flexor carpi radialis have their own synovial sheaths, and communications may exist among all the sheaths. The common flexor sheath does not extend into the fingers except for the fifth (the little finger). Here the sheath continues to the distal phalanx. For the second, third, and fourth digit tendons, there is a bare area before the synovial sheath encloses them again before entering the digits. From this area the lumbrical muscles take their origin.

The sheath around the flexor pollicis longus tendon extends from just proximal to the flexor retinaculum to the distal phalanx of the pollex (the thumb). See Fig. 3.34.

A penetrating injury to the digits can cause an infection. If it is within the synovial sheaths of the little finger or thumb, the infection may spread proximally to the palm by tracking through the sheath.

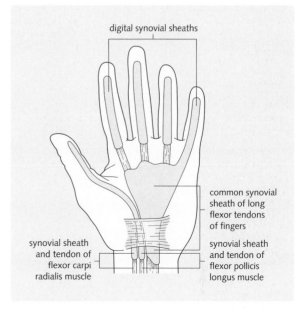

Fig. 3.34 Flexor synovial sheaths in the hand.

Long flexor tendons in the digits

The tendon of flexor digitorum superficialis bifurcates into two slips before inserting into the middle phalanx, and the flexor digitorum profundus runs between these slips to insert into the respective phalanges via delicate bands called vincula. As the tendons reach the metacarpophalangeal joints, they enter fibrous digital sheaths which are lined by the synovial sheaths. The fibrous flexor sheaths bind the tendons down to the finger. They are strong and thick over the phalanges but weak and loose over digit joints to allow movement (Fig. 3.35).

Nerves in the hand
Median nerve

The median nerve emerges from the carpal tunnel to enter the palm. Branches of the nerve in this region include:

- Muscular or recurrent branch to the muscles of the thenar eminence.
- Palmar digital nerves providing sensory innervation to the lateral three-and-a-half digits (including the nail bed and skin on the dorsum of the digit over the terminal phalanx) and motor supply to the first and second lumbricals.

51

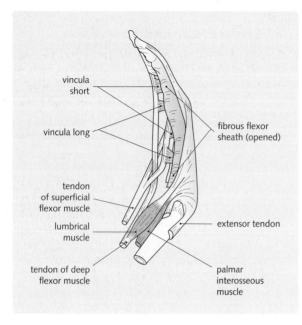

Fig. 3.35 Long flexor tendons of a finger and their vincula.

Damage to the median nerve, e.g., trauma to the wrist, results in loss of sensation to the lateral three-and-a-half digits and loss of function in the thumb. This is a very incapacitating injury that renders the entire upper limb almost functionless.

Ulnar nerve
The ulnar nerve and artery pass into the hand together, superficial to the flexor retinaculum but bound by fascia to its anterior surface. The nerve passes just medial to the pisiform bone. It divides into superficial and deep branches at the distal edge of the flexor retinaculum.

The superficial branch supplies palmaris brevis and palmar digital nerves to the medial one-and-a-half digits (including the skin over the dorsum of the distal phalanx).

The deep branch runs with the deep branch of the ulnar artery, and it supplies the hypothenar muscles, the medial lumbricals, all of the

interosseous muscles, the adductor pollicis, and the deep head of the flexor pollicis brevis.

See Fig. 3.30 for the cutaneous innervation of the palmar and dorsal surfaces of the hand.

Radial nerve
Although the radial nerve supplies no muscles in the hand, its superficial branch pierces the deep fascia near the dorsum of the wrist to provide sensation to the lateral two-thirds of the hand, the dorsum of the thumb, and the proximal areas of the lateral one and one-half digits (see Fig. 3.30).

Vessels of the hand
The radial artery slopes across the anatomic snuffbox overlying the scaphoid and trapezium and passes between the two heads of the first dorsal interosseous. It appears deep in the palm of the hand, emerging between the two heads of adductor pollicis and anastomosing with the deep branch of the ulnar artery to form the deep palmar arch. Palmar metacarpal arteries from the arch anastomose with the common palmar digital arteries of the superficial palmar arch.

The ulnar artery approaches the wrist between flexor digitorum superficialis and flexor carpi ulnaris. It enters the wrist with the ulnar nerve, superficial to the flexor retinaculum. In the hand it divides into two branches. One of these is the superficial palmar arch, from which common palmar digital arteries arise. The common digital arteries divide to form (proper) palmar digital arteries that enter the digits to supply the joints and phalanges. The other branch is the aforementioned deep palmar branch.

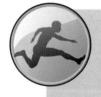

The radial pulse can be felt at the wrist, lateral to the flexor carpi radialis tendon, where the artery lies on the distal end of the radius.

Palmar spaces
The medial palmar or oblique septum from the palmar aponeurosis to the third metacarpal divides

the central part of the palm into two fascial spaces: the thenar space lies laterally and the midpalmar space lies medially.

These spaces contain the palmar muscles, tendons, vessels, and nerves in loose connective tissue and fat. Deep infections can spread to these spaces.

Nails

These lie on the dorsal surface of the distal phalanges, and they are plates of tightly packed, cornified epithelial cells. The uncornified epithelium on which the nail plate lies is called the nailbed. Both are supplied by the proper palmar vessels and nerves.

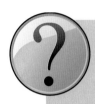

- Describe the superficial veins of the upper limb.
- Describe the lymphatic drainage of the upper limb.
- Describe the bones and joints of the pectoral girdle.
- Discuss the anatomy of the shoulder joint.
- What are the components and actions of the rotator cuff muscles?
- List the movements of the shoulder joint and the muscles causing them.
- List the boundaries and contents of the axilla.
- Draw the formation of the brachial plexus, including its roots, trunks, divisions, cords, and branches.
- Name the muscles and their nerve supply that are involved in elbow flexion and extension.
- Describe the vessels of the arm and their branches.
- List the boundaries and contents of the cubital fossa.
- Describe the elbow joint.
- Discuss the muscles involved in wrist and digit movement.
- Describe the branches of the median nerve in the forearm.
- Outline the boundaries and contents of the anatomic snuffbox.
- Describe the sensory and motor deficits that would occur if the radial nerve were severed (1) at the elbow and (2) at the wrist.
- Describe the sensory and motor deficits that would occur if the ulnar nerve were severed (1) at the elbow and (2) at the wrist.
- Describe the sensory and motor deficits that would occur if the median nerve were severed (1) at the elbow and (2) at the wrist.
- Describe the dorsal digital expansion and how the action of the muscles contributing to it result in extension and/or flexion at the DIP, PIP, and MCP joints.
- Outline the cutaneous nerve supply of the hand.
- Describe the organization of the synovial sheaths in the palm and the digits.
- Outline the carpal tunnel and the structures passing through it.
- Discuss the movements of the thumb and the muscles producing each movement.

4. The Thorax

Regions and components of the thorax

The thorax lies between the neck and the abdomen.

The thoracic cavity contains the heart, lungs, great vessels, trachea, and esophagus. The lungs lie laterally in the pleural cavities, and the other structures lie in a central compartment called the mediastinum.

The thoracic skeleton is formed by the thoracic vertebrae, the ribs, the costal cartilages, and the sternum. It protects the contents of the thoracic cavity and some abdominal contents (e.g., the liver and spleen).

Superiorly the thorax communicates with the neck through the thoracic inlet. Inferiorly the diaphragm separates the thorax from the abdominal cavity.

Surface anatomy and superficial structures

Bony landmarks

The bony landmarks of the thorax are illustrated in Fig. 4.1.

The bony sternum can be palpated in the midline of the thorax anteriorly. The manubrium is the widest and thickest of the three parts of the sternum. Its superior border has a palpable concavity called the jugular notch. The manubrium joins the body of the sternum at the manubriosternal joint (the sternal angle of Louis). The sternal angle is important clinically because the second costal cartilages articulate with the manubrium and the sternum at this level. Inferiorly, the body of the sternum articulates with the xiphoid process.

The first rib articulates with the manubrium via a synchondrosis. The second rib articulates with both the manubrium and the sternum at the sternal angle. Ribs 3–6 articulate with the sternum on each side via the costal cartilages. The costal margin runs from the xiphisternal junction and comprises the costal cartilages of ribs 7–10.

Posteriorly the spinous processes of the thoracic vertebrae are palpable inferior to the vertebra prominens—the spinous process of C7 vertebra.

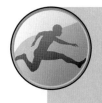

The manubriosternal joint is where the second costal cartilages articulate with it. This can be used as a reference point for counting the ribs.

Trachea, lungs, and pleurae

The trachea is palpable in the midline, above the suprasternal notch. It bifurcates behind the sternal angle (at the level of T5) into the right and left main bronchi.

The dome of the pleural cavity extends above the medial end of the clavicle into the thoracic inlet. The cavity is lined with a serous membrane called the parietal pleura (Fig. 4.2). The anterior border of the right pleura passes inferiorly behind the sternal angle to the xiphisternal joint. The anterior border of the left pleura follows a similar course, but at the level of the 4th costal cartilage it deviates laterally to approximately the costochondral angle and inferiorly to the 6th costal cartilage to form the cardiac notch. The lower border of the parietal pleura follows the costal margin, being at the level of the 8th rib in the midclavicular line, the 10th rib in the midaxillary line, and the 12th rib adjacent to the vertebral column. These are called the lines of pleural reflection.

Because the pleural cavity and the apex of the lung project upward into the thoracic inlet, they can be injured in wounds to the base of the neck.

The surface of the lungs is covered by visceral pleura, which is continuous with the parietal pleura at the root of the lung and which follows

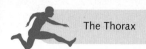
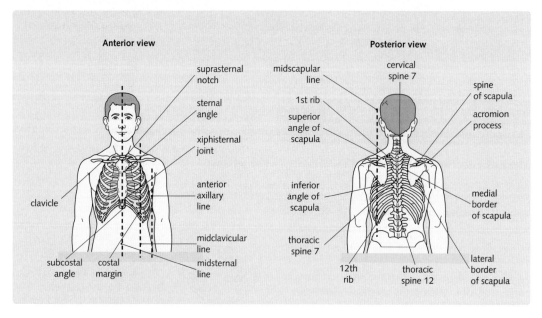

Fig. 4.1 Surface markings of the anterior and posterior thoracic walls.

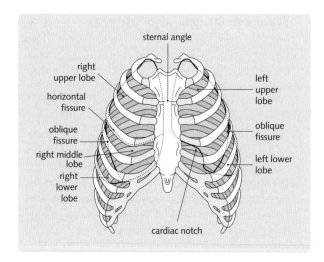

Fig. 4.2 Surface markings of the lungs.

the lines of reflection of the parietal pleura at mid-inspiration. These lines lie at the level of the 6th, 8th, and 10th ribs in the midclavicular line, midaxillary line, and adjacent to the vertebral column, respectively.

The space between the lower border of the pleura and lung is the costodiaphragmatic recess. In life, it is filled by the lungs in full inspiration. The spaces between the medial border of the parietal pleurae and the visceral pleurae covering the lungs at the lower third of the sternum are

called the costomediastinal recesses, and the one on the left is larger because of the cardiac notch.

Heart

The surface markings of the heart are outlined in Fig. 4.3. The apex of the heart is taken as lying approximately in the midclavicular line of the 5th intercostal space. This point takes into account differences in stature and children. The surface markings of the heart valves are illustrated in Fig. 4.4.

56

Outline of the surface landmarks of the heart	
Border	**Areas covered**
Superior border	From the superior border of the second left costal cartilage to the third right costal cartilage
Right border	From the third right costal cartilage to the sixth right costal cartilage, slightly convex
Left border	From the second left costal cartilage to the apex of the heart
Inferior border	From the sixth right costal cartilage to the apex
Apex	Lies in the fifth intercostal space, in the midclavicular line

Fig. 4.3 Outline of the surface landmarks of the heart.

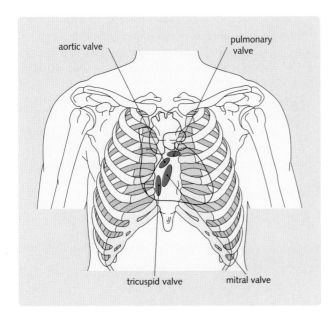

Fig. 4.4 Surface markings of the heart valves.

Great vessels

The aortic arch, a continuation of the ascending aorta, begins behind the sternal angle. It arches posteriorly and to the left of the vertebral column, where, again at the level of the sternal angle, the arch ends to become the descending (thoracic) aorta. The aortic arch, brachiocephalic trunk, and left common carotid and left subclavian arteries lie behind the manubrium. The brachiocephalic trunk bifurcates into the right common carotid and subclavian arteries behind the sternoclavicular joint (see Fig. 3.20).

The superior vena cava is formed behind the first right costal cartilage by the union of the brachiocephalic veins. The superior vena cava runs inferiorly along the right sternal border to enter the right atrium behind the third costal cartilage. The azygos vein joins the superior vena cava at the level of the second right costal cartilage.

The internal thoracic vessels run vertically downwards, posterior to the costal cartilages and 1 cm lateral to the sternal edge, as far as the 6th intercostal space. The arteries then divide into musculophrenic and superior epigastric arteries.

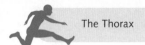
Diaphragm

The central tendon of the diaphragm lies behind the xiphisternal joint. In mid-respiration the right dome arches upwards to the upper border of the 5th rib in the midclavicular line; the left dome reaches only the lower border of the 5th rib.

Breasts

The breasts lie in the superficial fascia, mainly overlying the pectoralis major and serratus anterior muscles. They contain fat and mammary gland lobules, each of which is drained by a lactiferous duct that opens on the nipple. The nipple is the greatest prominence of the breast, and it is surrounded by a circular pigmented area called the areola. The mammary gland is attached to the dermis of the skin by substantial condensations of fibrous connective tissue called the suspensory ligaments of Cooper.

The base of the breast usually lies between the 2nd and 6th rib vertically, and from the midaxillary line to the lateral border of the sternum horizontally.

The blood supply to the breast is derived from the anterior intercostal arteries from the internal thoracic artery, the lateral thoracic and the thoracoacromial arteries, and the posterior intercostal arteries. Venous drainage is into the axillary and internal thoracic veins.

Lymph drains into the subareolar plexus and then into either axillary, deltopectoral, supraclavicular, or parasternal nodes.

Axillary nodes receive most of the lymphatic drainage of the breast (75%), particularly from the superior and lateral parts of the breast. Lymphatics from the inferior and medial part of the breast can drain into parasternal nodes and then via the bronchomediastinal lymph trunk into the lymphatics at the root of the neck (supraclavicular, deep cervical nodes).

Lymphatics may communicate with vessels from the opposite breast.

Carcinoma of the breast—the most common cancer affecting women—spreads via the lymphatics in many cases. A detailed knowledge of this drainage is required for appropriate treatment.

In advanced breast carcinoma, skin dimpling occurs due to tumor invasion and fibrosis, which cause a shortening of the suspensory ligaments.

The thoracic wall

The thoracic skeleton is formed by the sternum, the ribs and costal cartilages, and the thoracic vertebrae (Fig. 4.5).

Sternum

The sternum (breast bone) has three components:
- The manubrium is the upper part of the sternum. It articulates with the clavicles and with the 1st and upper part of the 2nd costal cartilages.
- The body of the sternum articulates with the manubrium at the manubriosternal joint at the level of the T4–T5 intervertebral disc superiorly, and with the xiphisternum inferiorly. These are fibrocartilaginous joints. Laterally the sternal body articulates with the 2nd to 7th costal cartilages via synovial joints.

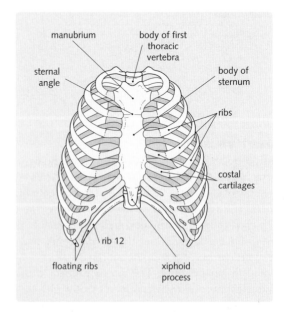

Fig. 4.5 Thoracic skeleton.

- The xiphoid process is the lowest part of the sternum, and it articulates with the sternum via the xiphisternal junction at the level of T9.

Ribs and costal cartilages

There are 12 pairs of ribs. They all articulate with a costal cartilage anteriorly via a hyaline cartilaginous joint. The upper seven ribs articulate directly with the sternum via their own costal cartilage. The 8th to 10th ribs have costal cartilages that are attached to each other and to the 7th anteriorly, and thence to the sternum. The 2nd–7th costal cartilages articulate with the sternum via synovial joints.

The 11th and 12th ribs have no anterior attachment for their costal cartilages.

Typical ribs (3rd–9th)

A typical rib has the following features (Fig. 4.6):

- It is a long, curved, flattened bone with a rounded superior border and a sharp thin inferior border with a costal groove paralleling it on the internal surface.
- It has a head with two demifacets for articulation with the numerically identical vertebral body and that of the vertebra immediately above.
- The neck separates the head and the tubercle.
- The tubercle has a facet for articulation with the transverse process of the corresponding vertebra.
- The shaft is thin, flat, and curved, with an angle at its point of greatest change in curvature.

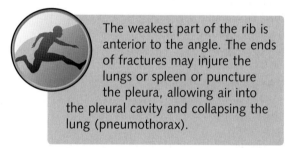

The weakest part of the rib is anterior to the angle. The ends of fractures may injure the lungs or spleen or puncture the pleura, allowing air into the pleural cavity and collapsing the lung (pneumothorax).

Atypical ribs

Fig. 4.7 shows the 1st rib and its relations in the thoracic inlet. This is the broadest, shortest, and

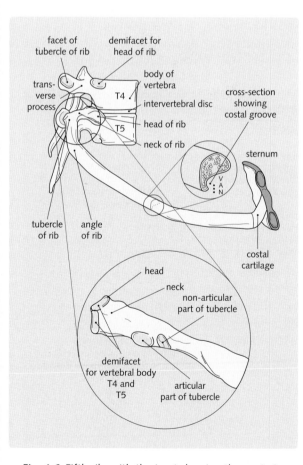

Fig. 4.6 Fifth rib, with the inset showing the posterior surface of the rib.

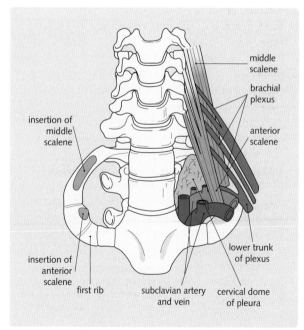

Fig. 4.7 First rib and its relations to the thoracic inlet.

59

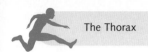

most sharply curved rib. It has a single facet on its head for articulation with the T1 vertebra only and a tubercle on the upper surface for attachment of the anterior scalene muscle. The subclavian artery and vein pass posterior and anterior to the tubercle, respectively. The second rib is very much like a typical rib except that its costal cartilage articulates anteriorly with both the manubrium and the sternum.

The 10th, 11th, and 12th ribs have one facet on the head for articulation with their own vertebra. The 11th and 12th ribs have no neck or tubercle.

A supernumerary cervical rib may compress the subclavian artery or the inferior trunk of the brachial plexus, causing ischemic pain and numbness in the area of distribution of the affected nerve.

Thoracic vertebrae

There are 12 thoracic vertebrae with their intervening intervertebral discs (see Chapter 2).

Openings into the thorax
Thoracic inlet (superior thoracic aperture)

The thoracic cavity communicates with the root of the neck via the thoracic inlet (see Fig. 4.7). The margins of the inlet include:
- T1 vertebra posteriorly.
- The pair of first ribs and their costal cartilage laterally.
- Superior border of the manubrium anteriorly.

The esophagus, trachea, and the apices of the lungs, together with various vessels and nerves that supply and drain the head, neck, and upper limbs, can be found in the inlet.

Thoracic outlet (inferior thoracic aperture)

The thoracic outlet lies between the thorax and the abdomen. It is bounded posteriorly by the 12th thoracic vertebra, posterolaterally by the 11th and 12th pairs of ribs, anteriorly by the costal margin and xiphoid process. It is closed by the diaphragm. Numerous structures pass through this opening (see Fig. 4.11).

Muscles of the thorax			
Name of muscle (nerve supply)	Origin	Insertion	Action
External intercostal (intercostal)	Inferior border of the rib above	Fibers run inferiorly and medially to the superior border of the rib below	All of the intercostal muscles assist in both inspiration during ventilation by maintaining the spaces between the ribs
Internal intercostal (intercostal)	Inferior border of the rib above	Fibers run inferiorly and laterally to the superior border of the rib below	
Innermost intercostal (intercostal)	Adjacent rib	Superior border of the 2nd or 3rd ribs below	
Transversus thoracis (intercostal)	Postrior surface of lower sternum	Internal surfaces of costal cartilages 2–6	Depresses ribs
Diaphragm (phrenic)	Two slips from posterior xiphoid process; internal sufaces and adjacent ribs of lower 6 costal cartilages; two crura or musculotendinous bundles from bodies of L1–L3 vertebrae; slips from medial and lateral arcuate ligaments	Central tendon	Important muscle of inspiration; increases vertical diameter of thorax by descent of central tendon

Fig. 4.8 Muscles of the thorax.

Intercostal spaces

The intercostal spaces lie between the ribs.

Below the skin and superficial fascia lie the three sets of intercostal muscles (Fig. 4.8). The innermost muscle layer is lined by the endothoracic fascia and the parietal pleura.

Intercostal nerves and vessels

The intercostal nerves are the anterior rami of the upper eleven thoracic spinal nerves. The anterior ramus of the 12th spinal nerve is the subcostal nerve.

The intercostal nerve runs in a plane between the parietal pleura and the posterior intercostal membrane, and at the angle of the rib, it passes forward between the innermost and internal intercostal muscles in the costal groove of the corresponding rib. At approximately the midaxillary line, a lateral cutaneous branch is given off, and near the sternum the intercostal nerve passes anteriorly between the costal cartilages to become the anterior cutaneous branch. The nerve has a collateral branch that runs along the upper border of the rib below.

The 1st–6th intercostal nerves supply the skin and parietal pleura and the intercostal muscles of their respective spaces. A large superior branch of the anterior ramus of the first spinal nerve passes to the brachial plexus. The second intercostal nerve gives rise to a large lateral cutaneous branch called the intercostobrachial nerve, which emerges from the 2nd intercostal space and enters the axilla to supply sensation to the medial surface of the arm. This is the only sensory nerve to the upper limb not derived from the brachial plexus.

The 7th–11th nerves cross the costal margin after giving off their lateral branches and supply the skin, peritoneum, and anterior abdominal wall muscles. The subcostal nerve runs beneath the diaphragm on the abdominal wall.

Fig. 4.9 shows the arterial supply to the thoracic wall.

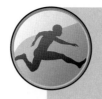 The intercostal neurovascular bundle running in the costal groove can be remembered as **VAN** (**v**ein, **a**rtery, **n**erve) from superior to inferior.

 When inserting an intercostal needle, introduce it into the middle of the space, avoiding the collateral branches of the neurovascular bundle and the structures in the costal groove.

Arterial supply to the thoracic wall		
Artery	**Origin**	**Distribution**
Anterior intercostal (spaces 1–6)	Internal thoracic artery	Intercostal muscles and parietal pleura
Antrior intercostal (spaces 7–9)	Musculoophrenic artery	
Posterior intercostal (all other spaces)	Superior intercostal artery, thoracic aorta	
Internal thoracic	Subclavian artery	Passes inferiorly just lateral to the sternum and terminates by dividing into the superior epigastric and musculophrenic arteries
Subcostal	Thoracic aorta	Courses under inferior border of the 12th rib to the muscles of adominal wall

Fig. 4.9 Arterial supply to the thoracic wall.

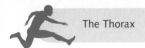

Diaphragm

The diaphragm is the primary muscle of respiration. It consists of a peripheral muscular part with numerous slips of origin (see Fig. 4.7) whose fibers converge radially on a central tendon, and it separates the thoracic and abdominal cavities. As viewed from the front, the diaphragm curves up into two domes, the right dome being higher than the left (Fig. 4.10) owing to the presence of the liver. When viewed from the side, it assumes an inverted J-shape.

Fig. 4.11 lists the openings in the diaphragm and the structures passing through them.

The blood and nerve supplies of the diaphragm are shown in Fig. 4.12.

To remember that the diaphragm has the phrenic nerve as its sole motor supply, use the mnemonic: C3, 4, 5 keeps the diaphragm alive.

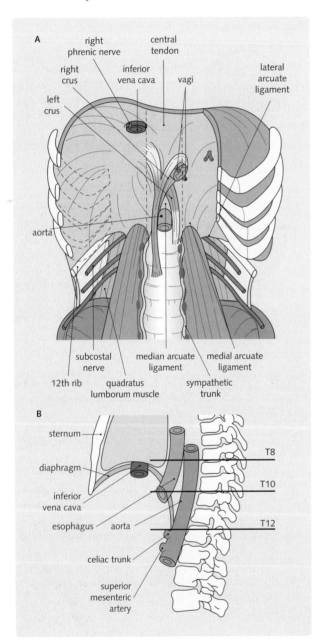

Fig. 4.10 Diaphragm as seen (A) from below (the anterior portion of the right side has been removed) and (B) as a sagittal section.

Diaphragmatic apertures and structures passing through them	
Opening	**Structures**
Aortic opening (behind the diaphragm at the level of T12)	Aorta, thoracic duct, and sometimes the azygos and hemiazygos veins
Esophageal opening (in the right crus of the diaphragm at the level of T10)	Esophagus, anterior and posterior vagal trunks, esophageal branches of the left gastric vessels and lymphatics
Vena caval opening (in the central tendon at the level of T8)	Inferior vena cava, right phrenic nerve, lymphatics
Small aperture in the right and left crura of the diaphragm	Greater and lesser splanchnic nerves
Behind the diaphragm	Sympathetic trunks and subcostal nerves
Sternocostal triangle between the sternal and costal attachments of the diaphragm	Superior epigastric vessels and lymphatics

Fig. 4.11 Diaphragmatic apertures and structures passing through them.

Nerves and vessels of the diaphragm	
Innervation	Motor supply: phrenic nerve (C3–C5); sensory supply: centrally by phrenic nerves (C3–C5), peripherally by intercostal nerves (T5–T11) and subcostal nerve (T12)
Arterial supply	Superior phrenic arteries, musculophrenic arteries, inferior phrenic arteries, pericardiophrenic arteries
Venous drainage	Musculophrenic and pericardiophrenic veins drain into internal thoracic vein; superior and inferior phernic veins drain into the inferior vena cava
Lymphatic drainage	Diaphragmatic lymph nodes drain to posterior mediastinal nodes eventually; superior lumbar, parasternal, and phrenic nodes; dense lymphatic plexus on inferior surface

Fig. 4.12 Nerves and vessels of the diaphragm.

The thoracic cavity

The thoracic cavity is filled laterally by the lungs and the pleural cavities. The median compartment separating the lungs and their pleurae is the mediastinum. This may be divided by a plane passing through the sternal angle (of Louis) and the T4–T5 intervertebral disc (Fig. 4.13). The superior mediastinum lies above this plane and contains the thymus, great vessels, trachea, esophagus, thoracic duct, vagus and phrenic nerves, sympathetic trunk, and recurrent laryngeal nerve.

The inferior mediastinum lies below the plane, and it is further subdivided into:

- The anterior mediastinum, lying between the pericardium and the sternum, which contains lymph nodes, fat, and remnants of the thymus.
- The middle mediastinum, which contains the pericardium, heart, and roots of the great vessels.
- The posterior mediastinum, lying between the pericardium and the vertebral column, which contains the esophagus, esophageal plexus, thoracic duct, sympathetic trunk, veins of the azygos system, and descending aorta.

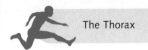
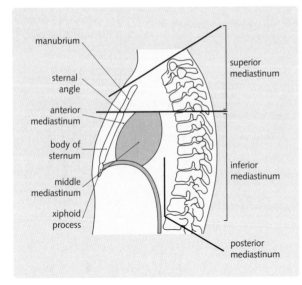

Fig. 4.13 Subdivisions of the mediastinum.

Fig. 4.14 shows the left and right sides of the mediastinum.

The mediastinum

Pericardium

The pericardium is a double-walled fibroserous sac that encloses the heart and the roots of the great vessels. It is divided into the fibrous pericardium and the two layers of the serous pericardium: the parietal, which lines the fibrous pericardium, and the visceral, which covers the heart and is also called the epicardium. The fibrous pericardium is a strong layer that limits the movement of the heart. It is attached to the central tendon of the diaphragm, the sternum, and the tunica adventitia of the great vessels. The parietal pericardium is continuous with the visceral pericardium around the roots of the great vessels.

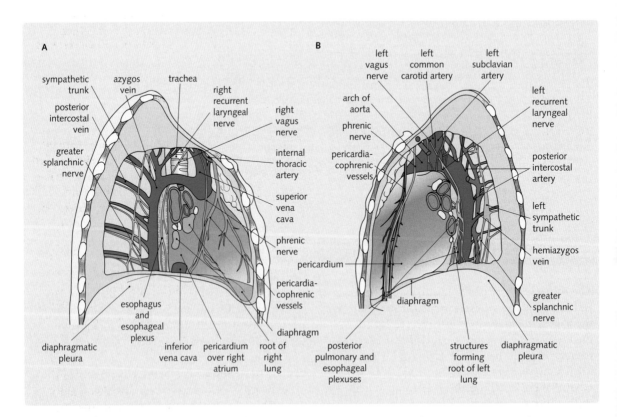

Fig. 4.14 (A) Right surface of the mediastinum and the right posterior thoracic wall. (B) Left surface of the mediastinum and the left posterior thoracic wall. Mediastinal pleura has been removed.

The nerve supply to the fibrous and parietal layer of the pericardium is by the phrenic nerves. However, the visceral layer has no somatic innervation, and so it is insensitive to pain. Therefore, pain from inflammation of the sac (pericarditis) is transmitted through the phrenic nerve and referred to the dermatomes of the shoulder through C3 and C4 spinal nerves.

The pericardium may be affected in many diseases, including tuberculosis and other infections, leading to inflammation and pericardial friction rub between the two visceral layers. Also, trauma to the heart may result in bleeding into the pericardium, which may compress the heart (cardiac tamponade); this is a true emergency—immediate drainage is needed if the patient is to survive.

Pericardial sinuses

The visceral layer of the serous pericardium around the entrances of the pulmonary veins creates a pocketlike recess posterior to the base of the heart, called the oblique sinus. A common sleeve of visceral pericardium around the aorta and pulmonary trunk and its separate reflection around the superior vena cava create the transverse sinus, which passes between them. This allows the arterial pole of the heart to be clamped separately during open heart surgery (see Fig. 4.15).

Heart

This is the muscular organ responsible for pumping blood throughout the body (Fig. 4.16). It lies free in the pericardium, connected only at its base to the great vessels.

The walls of the heart consist mainly of heart muscle (myocardium), lined internally by endocardium and externally by epicardium (visceral serous pericardium).

The heart has four chambers: the right and left atria and the right and left ventricles. The right side of the heart receives poorly oxygenated blood from the body and pumps it to the lungs, while the left side receives well-oxygenated blood from the lungs and pumps it throughout the remainder of the body.

Chambers of the heart
Right atrium

This chamber consists of the right atrium proper and an atrial appendage, the right auricle

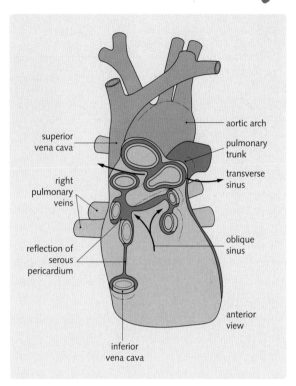

Fig. 4.15 Pericardial sinuses and reflections (the heart has been removed). Anterior view. (Adapted from Gray's Anatomy, 38th edn., edited by L.H. Bannister et al. Harcourt Brace and Co.)

(Fig. 4.17). There is a shallow, vertically oriented groove on the external surface of the atrium, called the sulcus terminalis, and a corresponding internal ridge, called the crista terminalis. The atrium posterior to the crista terminalis is smooth-walled, while the region anterior to it is ridged by rough muscles—the musculi pectinati.

The inferior vena cava opens into the inferior right atrium, while the superior vena cava enters superiorly, almost in a direct line above it. The opening of the coronary sinus, which brings blood from the cardiac veins, lies between the orifice of the inferior vena cava and the atrioventricular orifice.

Interatrial septum

This forms the posterior wall of the right atrium. In the lower part of the septum is a depression, called the fossa ovalis. This is the remnant of the foramen ovale and its valve in the fetal heart. The

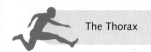

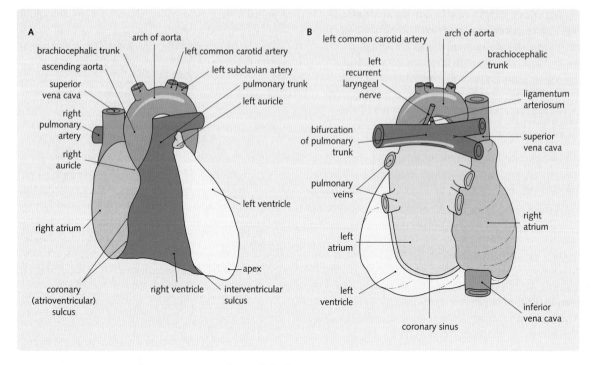

Fig. 4.16 Anterior (A) and posterior (B) surfaces of the heart.

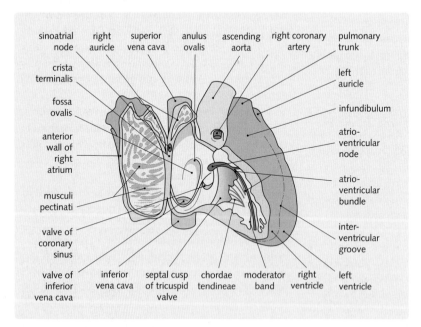

Fig. 4.17 Interior of right atrium and right ventricle.

limbus of the fossa ovalis is the raised margin surrounding the fossa.

Right ventricle

Blood enters the right ventricle via the atrioventricular orifice guarded by the right cuspid valve (Fig. 4.17), while blood flows out of the right ventricle via the pulmonary trunk with its pulmonary valve. The ventricle becomes funnel-shaped as it approaches the pulmonary orifice—this region is known as the infundibulum.

The tricuspid valve has three cusps (anterior, posterior, and septal), the bases of which are attached to a fibrous ring of the skeleton of the heart around the atrioventricular orifice.

The ventricular wall has many prominent muscular ridges, called trabeculae carneae. Some of these are specialized:

- Papillary muscles—attached to the ventricular wall and to the cusps of the tricuspid valve via fibrous cords, the chordae tendineae. Each cusp is attached to two of the three papillary muscles: anterior, posterior, and septal. The muscles contract to prevent the cusps from being everted into the atrium by pressure in the contracting ventricle.
- Moderator band or septomarginal trabecula—contains part of the conducting system of the heart and runs from the septal wall to near the apex of the ventricle.

The three cusps of the pulmonary valve—right, left, and anterior—are attached to the arterial wall at their lower margins and resemble vest pockets. The 'pockets' between the cusp and the wall of the artery collect blood that backflows after being ejected from the ventricle.

Left atrium
The left atrium forms most of the base of the heart. It consists of a main cavity and an atrial appendage, the left auricle. The four pulmonary veins enter through the posterior wall. The left atrioventricular orifice is guarded by the bicuspid mitral valve.

The posterior half of this chamber, into which the pulmonary veins enter, has smooth walls. The anterior portion, continuous with the auricle, is ridged by musculi pentinati.

Left ventricle
The left ventricle is responsible for pumping blood throughout all the body except the lungs. Consequently, its walls are three times thicker than those of the right ventricle, and pressures in this chamber are up to six times greater.

There are well-developed trabeculae carneae and two large papillary muscles, anterior and posterior. The smooth-walled, nonmuscular region of the ventricle below the aorta is the aortic vestibule.

The mitral valve or bicuspid valve guards the left atrioventricular orifice. It is bicuspid (anterior and posterior), with attached chordae tendineae similar to the tricuspid valve.

The three-cusped aortic valve is similar to the pulmonary valve. Behind each cusp—anterior, left, and right—lies an aortic sinus. The orifice of the right coronary artery is in the aortic wall behind the right cusp, while the orifice of the left coronary artery is behind the left cusp.

The interventricular septum is an obliquely oriented partition between the two ventricles that is largely muscular. Because of higher pressure on the left side, it bulges into the right ventricle. Superiorly, where the septum is continuous with the fibrous ring, it is thinner and more fibrous—this is the membranous part of the septum. Above the attachment of the cusp, this membranous part actually separates the right atrium from the right ventricle.

Skeleton of the heart
The muscular fibers of the two atria and two ventricles are anchored to a pair of fibrous rings around the atrioventricular orifices and partial rings or coronets around the aortic and pulmonary orifices. Left and right fibrous trigones are formed by the connections between these rings. The fibrous rings separate the muscle fibers of the atria and ventricles, with the atrioventricular conducting system forming the only physiologic connection between the atria and ventricles.

The bases of the cusps of the atrioventricular valves and the membranous part of the atrioventricular septum are also attached to the fibrous skeleton.

Blood supply of the heart
Fig. 4.18 illustrates the blood supply of the heart. The ascending aorta has two branches, which arise from aortic sinuses. These branches are the right and left coronary arteries. Both run in the coronary groove.

The right coronary artery in 60% of individuals supplies the sinoatrial node and in 90% of individuals supplies the atrioventricular node. The atrioventricular bundle and its right terminal branch are supplied by the right coronary artery the majority of the time. The left terminal branch is supplied by both right and left coronary arteries.

Left and right dominance of the heart is a reference to the coronary artery from which the

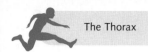

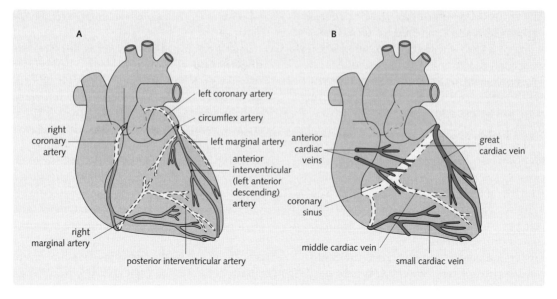

Fig. 4.18 Blood supply of the heart: (A) coronary arteries; (B) cardiac veins.

posterior interventricular branch arises. Right dominance is more common: the posterior interventricular branch arises from the right coronary artery.

Narrowing of the coronary arteries (coronary artery disease [CAD]), usually due to an atherosclerotic process of lipid deposition in their walls, gives rise to conditions such as angina pectoris and myocardial infarction. CAD is the most common cause of death in the Western world. The anterior interventricular artery is most commonly affected, followed by the right coronary artery.

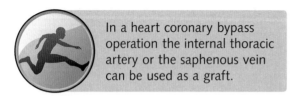

In a heart coronary bypass operation the internal thoracic artery or the saphenous vein can be used as a graft.

Venous drainage of the heart
Most of the venous blood in the heart drains from cardiac veins into the coronary sinus, which lies in the posterior atrioventricular groove. The great cardiac vein drains the area supplied by the left coronary artery and is the main tributary of the coronary sinus, which opens into the right atrium.

The small and middle cardiac veins drain the area supplied by the right coronary artery and also empty into the coronary sinus.

The remaining blood is returned to the heart via the anterior cardiac veins to the right atrium and other small veins (venae cordis minimae) that open directly into the heart chambers.

Conducting system of the heart
The heart contracts rhythmically at about 70 beats per minute.

The sinoatrial node (pacemaker) is a small collection of modified muscle fibers and lies at the superior end of the sulcus terminalis near the junction of the superior vena cava and the right atrium. Impulses generated here are transmitted throughout the atria, causing them to contract, and to the atrioventricular node, which lies in the atrial septum just above the attachment of the septal cusp of the tricuspid valve and the entrance of the coronary sinus. Impulses from the atrioventricular node are conducted to the atrioventricular bundle.

The atrioventricular bundle divides into two branches at the junction of the membranous and muscular parts of the interventricular septum, such that the right and left bundles straddle the muscular part of the septum.

• The right branch conducts the impulse to the muscle of the right ventricle, the interventricular septum, and, via the moderator band, to the anterior papillary muscle.

- The left branch descends on the left side of the septum and passes down on the left side beneath the endocardium. Near its origin it divides into several branches that supply the interventricular septum and the left ventricle.

Fig. 4.19 details the nerve supply of the heart.

Referred pain from a myocardial infarction is transmitted by afferent fibers back through the cardiac branches of the cervical sympathetic trunk. Afferent fibers enter the spinal cord of the upper five thoracic nerves, and pain is referred to dermatomes over the shoulder and upper limb.

Outline of the nerve supply to the heart		
Nerve type	Origin	Action
Sympathetic nerves (preganglionic)	Cervical and superior thoracic sympathetic trunk to the cardiac plexus	Increase the rate and force of contraction and of impulse conduction
Parasympathetic nerves (preganglionic)	Vagus nerves to the cardiac plexus	Reduce the rate and force of contraction, constrict coronary arteries

Fig. 4.19 Outline of the nerve supply of the heart.

Aorta and its branches in the thorax		
Artery	Course and origin	Branches
Ascending aorta	Originates from the left ventricle, ascends and becomes the aortic arch at the level of the sternal angle	Right and left coronary arteries
Aortic arch	Arches posteriorly to the left of the trachea and the esophagus and continues as the descending aorta	Brachiocephalic trunk, left common carotid artery, left subclavian artery
Descending aorta	Descends to the left of the vertebral column, moves anterior to reach the midline, and leaves the thorax by passing behind the diaphragm at T12	Posterior intercostal arteries, subcostal arteries and visceral branches
Bronchial (1–2)	Arise from the anterior surface of the descending aorta	To bronchi and visceral pleura
Esophageal (4–5)	Arise from the anterior surface of the descending aorta	To esophagus
Superior phrenic (variable in number)	Arise from the descending aorta	To diaphragm
Posterior intercostals	Arise from the posterior surface of the descending aorta	To intercostal muscles and thoracic wall via lateral and anterior cutaneous branches

Fig. 4.20 Aorta and its branches in the thorax.

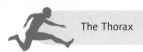

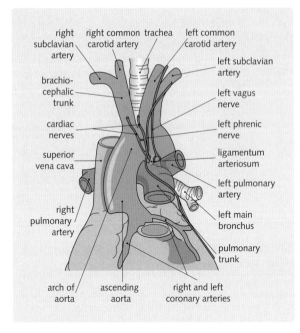

right subclavian artery — right common carotid artery — trachea — left common carotid artery

left subclavian artery

brachio-cephalic trunk

left vagus nerve

cardiac nerves

left phrenic nerve

superior vena cava

ligamentum arteriosum

right pulmonary artery

left pulmonary artery

left main bronchus

pulmonary trunk

arch of aorta — ascending aorta — right and left coronary arteries

Fig. 4.21 Aorta and pulmonary trunk.

Great vessels of the thorax

Fig. 4.20 outlines the thoracic aorta and its branches. Fig. 4.21 shows the aortic arch and pulmonary trunk.

Note that the phrenic nerve passes anterior to the lung root. The vagus nerve passes posterior to the lung root.

Pulmonary trunk

This vessel transports deoxygenated blood from the right ventricle to the lungs.

The entire course of the pulmonary trunk lies within the pericardial sac, and it bifurcates into the right and left pulmonary arteries in the concavity of the arch of the aorta. Just outside the pericardium, the left pulmonary artery is connected to the arch of the aorta by the ligamentum arteriosum (see Fig. 4.21). It is a fibrous remnant of the ductus arteriosus, which in the fetus conducts blood from the pulmonary trunk to the aorta, bypassing the lungs.

Superior vena cava

The superior vena cava drains blood from all of the structures above the diaphragm except the heart

and lungs. It also receives blood from the azygos vein, which passes over the root of the right lung to drain to the superior vena cava, before it enters the pericardial sac. The azygos veins drain blood from the posterior intercostal (2–12), bronchial, pericardial, mediastinal, esophageal, subcostal, and ascending lumbar veins, along with the vertebral venous plexus (see Fig. 4.23). Thus, the superior vena cava drains thoracic structures indirectly. The superior vena cava empties into the right atrium.

Inferior vena cava

The inferior vena cava pierces the central tendon of the diaphragm at the level of the T8 vertebra, and almost immediately it enters the right atrium.

Fig. 4.22 shows the superior and inferior venae cavae and their main tributaries.

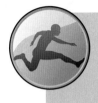

The azygos, accessory hemiazygos, and hemiazygos veins offer an alternative venous blood flow route from thoracic, abdominal, and back regions.

Pulmonary veins

Two pulmonary veins leave each lung at its root, carrying oxygenated blood to the left atrium of the heart.

Azygos system of veins

The azygos system of veins is variable in its origin, course, and tributaries. Fig. 4.23 shows a typical azygos system of veins and the thoracic duct.

Nerves of the thorax

Fig. 4.24 lists the main nerves of the thorax (see also Fig. 4.14).

Thoracic sympathetic trunk

The sympathetic trunks follow a paravertebral course, descending on the front of the heads of the ribs. By the time they leave the thorax by passing behind the median arcuate ligaments, they lie over the bodies of the vertebrae.

There is usually a ganglion for each thoracic spinal nerve, but the first ganglion usually merges with the inferior cervical ganglion to form the stellate ganglion. The last ganglion usually provides

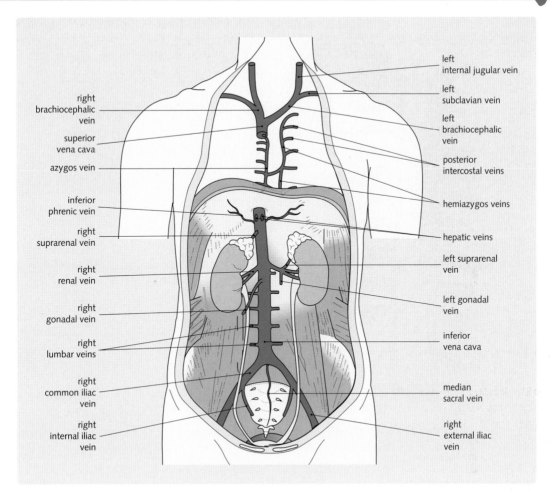

Fig. 4.22 Superior and inferior venae cavae and their main tributaries.

innervation to both the 11th and 12th nerves, for a total of 11 ganglia.

White and gray rami communicantes from the sympathetic trunk communicate with the thoracic spinal nerves.

The sympathetic trunk gives rise to the greater, lesser, and least splanchnic nerves. The greater nerve is formed by branches from the 5th to 9th ganglia. The lesser nerve is formed by branches from the 9th and 10th ganglia, and the least nerve is a branch of the lowest ganglion. These pass into the abdomen behind the diaphragm. The greater and lesser splanchnic nerves contain preganglionic fibers that synapse in the celiac ganglion and supply abdominal structures. The fibers in the least splanchnic nerve usually synapse in the renal plexus.

Lymphatic drainage of the thorax

Fig. 4.25 shows the lymphatic drainage of the thoracic cavity.

The thoracic duct (see Fig. 4.23) receives lymph from:
• The lower half of the body.
• The left side of the thorax.
• The left side of the head and neck, and the left upper limb, via the left jugular and subclavian lymph trunks, respectively.

It empties into the venous system near the union of the left internal jugular and the left subclavian veins. The lymphatics receiving lymph from the right side of the thorax, the right side of the head and neck, and the right upper limb drain into the right jugular and subclavian trunks, respectively.

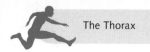
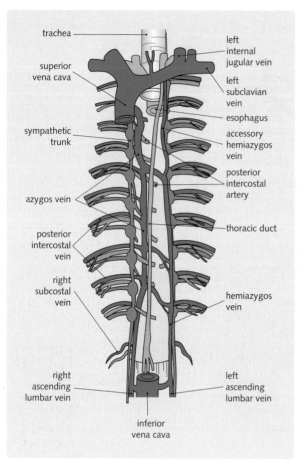

Fig. 4.23 Azygos system of veins and the thoracic duct.

These vessels drain into the veins of the same name, either independently or as a short single trunk, the right lymphatic trunk.

Thymus

This is the major organ responsible for the maturation of T lymphocytes, which is necessary for the development of immunologic competence. It is a large bilobed organ at birth, lying in the superior and anterior divisions of the mediastinum, anterior to the great vessels and posterior to the mediastinum. The gland involutes after puberty.

Trachea

The trachea (Fig. 4.26) commences in the neck, at the lower border of the cricoid cartilage. It passes into the superior mediastinum, anterior to the esophagus and close to the midline. At the sternal angle, the trachea bifurcates into the right and left main bronchi. The right main bronchus is shorter, wider, and more vertical than the left—foreign bodies are therefore more likely to lodge in this bronchus or one of its branches.

Esophagus

This organ is a fibromuscular tube that commences as a continuation of the laryngopharynx at the level of the C6 vertebra. In the thorax the esophagus descends between the trachea and the vertebral column. It then inclines to the left, passes through the diaphragm at the level of the T10 vertebra, and after 1–2 cm enters the stomach. Fibers from the right crus of the diaphragm form a sling around the esophagus.

The upper esophageal sphincter is part of the inferior constrictor of the pharynx and lies at the level of cricopharyngeus. This is the first narrowed part of the esophagus, with the others occurring

Nerves of the thorax	
Nerve (origin)	**Course and distribution**
Vagus, X (medulla oblongata)	Enters superior mediastinum posterior to sternoclavicular joint and brachiocephalic vein; right vagus descends anterior to the right subclavian artery and the left between the left common carotid and left subclavian arteries; supplies pulmonary plexus, esophageal plexus, and cardiac plexus
Phrenic (anterior rami of C3–C5)	Enters superior mediastinum between the subclavian artery and the origin of the brachiocephalic vein, passing anterior to the root of the lung between mediastinal pleura and pericardium; descends on the lateral aspect of the pericardium to supply motor and sensory innervation to diaphragm and sensory innervation to mediastinal pleura, pericardium, diaphragmatic pleura, and diaphragmatic peritoneum
Intercostal nerves (anterior rami of T1–T11)	Run between internal and innermost layers of intercostal muscles and supply skin, muscles and parietal pleura of intercostal spaces. Lower intercostal nerves also supply skin, muscles, and peritoneum of anterior abdominal wall
Subcostal (anterior ramus of T12)	Follows inferior border of 12th rib and passes into abdominal wall to supply the T12 dermatome and muscles
Recurrent laryngeal (X)	Loops around subclavian artery on right and arch of aorta on left and ascends in tracheoesophageal groove; supplies intrinsic muscles of larynx (except cricothyroid) and sensation inferior to level of vocal folds
Cardiac plexus (X and sympathetic trunks)	Fibers from posterior to the aorta and pulmonary trunk pass along coronary arteries to sinoatrial node; parasympathetic fibers reduce heart rate and force of contraction; sympathetic fibers increase rate and contraction force
Pulmonary plexus (X and sympathetic trunks)	Plexus forms on root of lung and extends along branches of bronchi; parasympathetic fibers constrict bronchioles, sympathetic fibers dilate them
Esophageal (X and sympathetic trunks)	Vagus and sympathetic nerves form a plexus around esophagus to supply muscle and glands of esophagus; above the diaphragm plexus gives rise to anterior and posterior vagal trunks

Fig. 4.24 Nerves of the thorax.

where it is in contact with the aorta, where it is crossed by left main bronchus, and where it pierces the diagphragm.

Fig. 4.27 outlines the blood supply, lymphatic drainage, and nerve supply of the esophagus.

Pleurae and lungs

Pleurae

The pleurae are two serous membranes that surround the lungs: the parietal and the visceral (Fig. 4.28).

The parietal pleura lines the thoracic wall (costal pleura), the thoracic surface of the diaphragm (diaphragmatic pleura), and the lateral aspect of the mediastinum (mediastinal pleura). At the thoracic inlet, it arches over the lungs as the cervical pleura, which lies above the clavicle at this point.

The visceral pleura is firmly adherent to the lungs, completely investing the outer surface of the lung and invaginating into the fissures of the lungs.

The two layers are continuous with each other at the root of the lung. Inferior to the root of the lung, this continuity exists as a double layer that contains no lung tissue but extends between the lung and mediastinum, the pulmonary ligament.

The pleural cavity is a potential space that exists between the two pleural layers. In a healthy person, the pleural cavity is empty except for a lubricating layer of pleural fluid. The pleural fluid maintains the surface tension that keeps the visceral pleura applied to the parietal pleura on the internal thoracic wall. This ensures that the lungs expand when the thorax expands.

Where the parietal pleura is reflected off the diaphragm onto the thoracic wall, a recess is formed that is not filled with lung except in deep

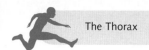

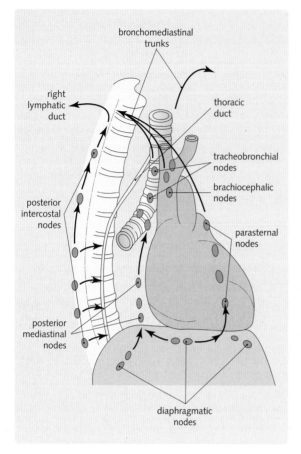

Fig. 4.25 Lymphatic drainage of the thoracic cavity.

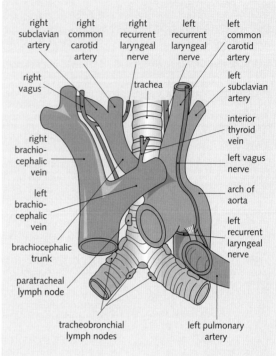

Fig. 4.26 Trachea and its main relations anteriorly and laterally.

	Blood and nerve supply and lympathic drainage of the esophagus		
	Upper esophagus	Middle esophagus	Lower esophagus
Arterial supply	Inferior thyroid artery	Esophageal branches of the aorta	Left gastric artery
Venous drainage	Inferior thyroid vein	Azygos and hemiazygos veins	Esophageal tributaries of the left gastric veins, which drain finally into the portal vein
Nerve supply	Recurrent laryngeal nerves and sympathteic fibers from cell bodies in the middle cervical ganglion running on the inferior thyroid artery	Parasympathetic fibers from the accessory nerves (CNXI) and from the vagus nerve (CNX) via the esophageal plexus; sympathetic fibers from the cervical and thoracic sympathetic trunks and abdominal splanchnic nerves	
Lymphatic drainage	Deep cervical nodes near the origin of the inferior thyroid artery	Tracheobronchial and posterior mediastinal nodes	Left gastric nodes of the celiac group

Fig. 4.27 Blood and nerve supply and lymphatic drainage of the esophagus.

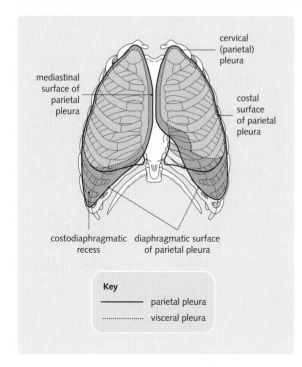

Fig. 4.28 Pleurae.

Nerve supply of the pleura	
Pleura	**Nerve supply**
Costal	Segmentally by the intercostal nerves
Mediastinal	The phrenic nerve
Diaphragmatic	The phrenic nerve centrally, the lower five intercostal nerves peripherally
Visceral	Autonomic nerve supply from the pulmonary plexus

Fig. 4.29 Nerve supply of the pleura.

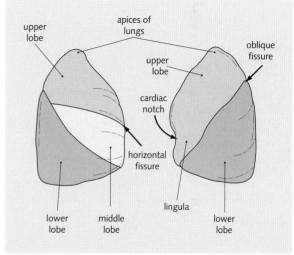

Fig. 4.30 Surface of the lungs.

inspiration. This is the costodiaphragmatic recess. A similar recess is formed between the thoracic wall and mediastinum (costomediastinal recess).

The nerve supply of the pleura is described in Fig. 4.29. The visceral pleura has no somatic innervation, and it is, therefore, insensitive to pain.

Blood supply of the pleurae
The parietal pleura is supplied by the intercostal arteries and branches of the internal thoracic artery. Venous drainage and lymphatic drainage are similarly shared.

The visceral pleura is supplied by the bronchial arteries. It shares venous and lymphatic drainage with the lung.

Endothoracic fascia
This is a very thin layer of loose connective tissue that binds the parietal pleura to the thoracic wall. It includes the suprapleural membrane, a distinct layer that covers the dome of the parietal pleura where it projects into the root of the neck and that limits bulging of the lung into the neck.

Lungs
The lungs in life are light, spongy, and elastic. The surface changes from a pink color at birth to a

mottled darker color in later life because of deposition of carbon particles from atmospheric pollution. This is more pronounced in city-dwellers and smokers.

In the pleural cavities each lung is attached at its root, where bronchi, vessels, and nerves enter and leave.

Surfaces and borders of the lungs
These are indicated in Figs. 4.30 and 4.31. Each lung has an apex that projects into the neck about 1 cm above the clavicle, a base that lies against the diaphragm, a costal surface, and a mediastinal surface.

75

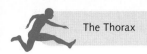

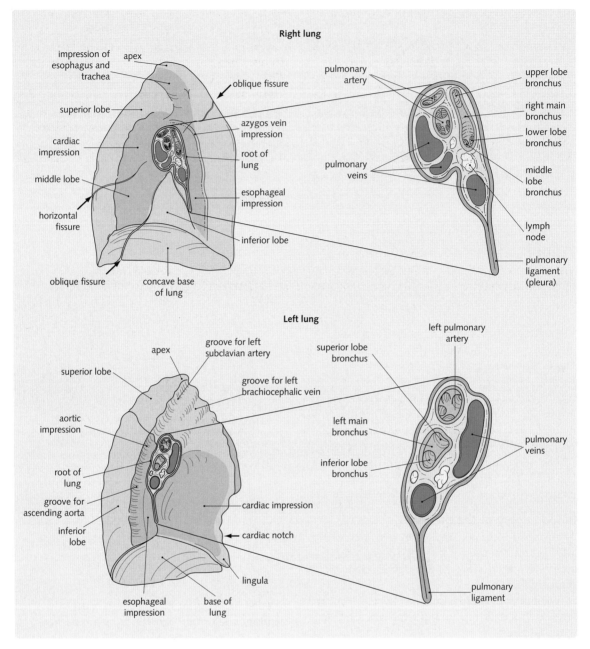

Fig. 4.31 Medial aspect of the right and left lungs and contents of their roots. Impressions are only seen in fixed lungs.

The hilum (root) of the lung (see Fig. 4.31) is found on the mediastinal surface where the bronchi and neurovascular bundles enter the lungs.

Lobes and fissures

The right lung has three lobes, and the left lung has two, created by the oblique and horizontal fissures.

The oblique fissure of the lungs runs from the level of the spinous process of T2 posteriorly to the sixth costal cartilage anteriorly. This line corresponds to the medial border of the scapula when the arm is raised above the shoulder. The horizontal fissure, which is present only in the right lung, extends from the oblique fissure at the midaxillary line along the fourth rib and costal cartilage anteriorly.

The anterior border of the left lung has a deep cardiac notch. The notch often creates a thin tongue-like process of the superior lobe called the lingual, which overlies the pericardium and slides in and out of the costomediastinal recess.

Bronchi and bronchopulmonary segments

The trachea divides into the right and left main bronchi. These are fibromuscular tubes reinforced by cartilaginous plates and lined by respiratory epithelium.

In the lung, the main bronchus divides into secondary (lobar) bronchi, upper, middle, and lower on the right and upper and lower on the left, which in turn divide into tertiary (segmental) bronchi. The latter supply the bronchopulmonary segments, which are the functional units of the lung (Fig. 4.32).

Bronchopulmonary segments are wedge-shaped, with the base lying peripherally and the apex lying toward the root of the lungs. There are 10 segments in the right lung and 8–10 in the left lung, depending on the combining of some

segments. Each segment has its own segmental bronchus, segmental pulmonary artery, lymphatic vessels, bronchial arteries and veins, and autonomic nerves. The veins lie between adjacent segments. Within each segment the segmental bronchus repeatedly subdivides and reduces in size until the cartilage in the walls disappears. The airway is now called a terminal bronchiole. These subdivide and eventually give rise to alveolar sacs, lined by alveoli. Alveoli have walls of a single-cell thickness, with no muscle. By the age of 8 years, a child has approximately 300 million alveoli. The thinness of their walls and the huge amount of surface area promote the efficient exchange of gas.

> The basal superior bronchopulmonary segment runs directly posteriorly at 90 degrees to the bronchial tree. In supine patients, bronchial secretions can drain into this segment, leading to pneumonia in the upper lobe.

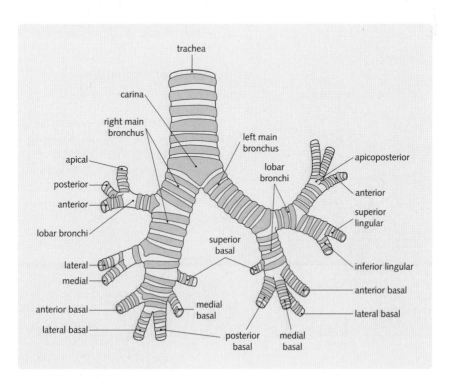

Fig. 4.32 The bronchial tree of the lung.

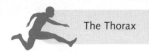

Nerve supply of the lungs

Sympathetic and parasympathetic nerves from the pulmonary plexuses, which lie anterior and posterior to the lung roots, supply the smooth muscle of the bronchial tree, the vessels, and the mucous membrane.

Blood supply of the lungs

The lungs have a dual blood supply:

- Bronchial arteries from the thoracic aorta supply the bronchi, the connective tissue of the lung, and the visceral pleura. Bronchial veins drain blood from lung tissue near the root and return it to the azygos system of veins.
- Pulmonary arteries transport deoxygenated blood to the alveolar capillaries. The pulmonary veins return oxygenated blood to the heart along with blood from lung tissue distal to the root and from the visceral pleura.

There are anastomoses between the pulmonary and bronchial circulations.

Pulmonary thromboembolism is a blockage of the pulmonary vasculature by a blood clot, leading to impaired gas exchange and increased vascular resistance. It can be asymptomatic, or its

symptoms can mimic those of other conditions. Thus it has an untreated mortality rate of 30%. Over 90% of the time these clots originate in the deep veins in the legs and pelvis and result from injury or inactivity.

Lymphatic drainage of the lungs

Fig. 4.33 illustrates the lymphatic drainage of the lungs.

Bronchogenic carcinoma or lung cancer accounts for 28% of all cancer-related deaths in the USA. It usually spreads via the lymphatics, and it has a poor prognosis. An understanding of the anatomy and lymphatic drainage is essential for planning treatment and assessing the prognosis of these tumors.

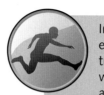 In bronchogenic carcinoma, enlarging of the tracheobronchial nodes can widen the tracheal bifurcation, and also it may involve the left recurrent laryngeal nerve, paralyzing the muscles of the left vocal fold and causing voice hoarseness and weakness.

Mechanics of respiration

Respiration consists of an inspiratory and an expiratory phase (Fig. 4.34).

Chronic obstructive pulmonary disease (COPD) is the leading cause of death, disability, and illness in the USA. Patients with COPD, which includes asthma and emphysema, can be seen using their accessory muscles of respiration, which include the sternocleidomastoid, pectoralis, scalene, and anterior abdominal muscles.

 If the intercostal muscles are paralyzed (e.g., in a nerve injury), they become relaxed. This is seen on inspiration when the muscles are sucked in and on expiration when the muscles bulge out.

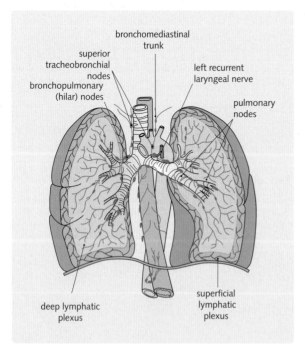
Fig. 4.33 Lymphatic drainage of the lungs.

Movements and muscles involved in respiration		
Movements	**Effect**	**Muscles involved**
Quiet inspiration	Increased vertical diameter	Diaphragm contracts
Quiet inspiration	Increased anteroposterior diameter	The upper intercostal muscles contract to elevate the upper ribs at their sternal ends toward the first rib, and this pushes the sternum forward—known as the pump handle movement
Quiet inspiration	Increased transverse diameter	The intercostal muscles contract, raising the ribs along an anteroposterior axis that runs through the costochondral joint (anteriorly) and costovertebral joint (posteriorly). The ribs are raised upward and and outward in a bucket handle movement
Forced inspiration	Increase of all three diameters	In addition to the diaphragm contracting, the anterior and middle scalenes elevate the first rib, the posterior scalene elevates the second rib, and the sternocleidomastoid, sternothyroid, and sternohyoid elevate the ribs and the manubrium. The intercostal muscles elevate the ribs. Quadratus lumborum fixes the twelfth rib. This allows a forceful diaphragmatic contraction. The erector spinae muscles arch the back and increase the thoracic volume. With the humerus and scapula fixed by the trapezius, rhomboid, and levator scapulae muscles, the pectoral and serratus anterior muscles raise the ribs
Quiet expiration	Decrease of all three diameters	Controlled relaxation of the intercostal and diaphragmatic muscles decreases intrathoracic volume and increases intra-abdominal pressure, and the elastic recoil of the lungs expels most air
Forced expiration	Decrease of all three diameters	Contraction of the anterior abdominal wall muscles depresses the ribs and increases intra-abdominal pressure to force the diaphragm upward. The diaphragm, scalene, sternocleidomastoid, sternothyroid, and sternohyoid muscles relax. The intercostal muscles relax to lower the ribs but maintain the space between the ribs

Fig. 4.34 Movements and muscles involved in respiration.

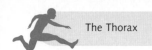

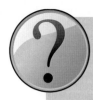

- Draw the surface features of the lung.
- Describe the lines of pleural reflection and their significance.
- Draw the surface projections of the heart and its valves.
- Describe where the valves are auscultated.
- What are the surface projections of the great vessels?
- Describe the lymphatic drainage of the breast and its importance.
- Describe the differences between typical and atypical ribs.
- List the boundaries of the thoracic inlet and outlet.
- Describe a typical intercostal space and its contents.
- Describe the anatomy of the diaphragm, including structures passing through and peripheral to it and its vascular and nerve supply.
- List the divisions of the mediastinum and their contents.
- Describe the pericardium and how the pericardial sinuses are formed.
- Describe the internal structure of the heart chambers.
- Define the blood supply to the heart, including left/right dominance and venous drainage.
- Describe the thoracic sympathetic trunk and the thoracic splanchnic nerves.
- Discuss the lymphatic drainage of the thorax.
- Discuss the anatomy of the esophagus, including its course, innervation, and blood supply.
- Describe the azygos system and its significance to the venous drainage of the thorax.
- Describe the trachea, the location of the tracheal bifurcation, and its relationship to surrounding structures.
- Describe the relationship of other structures to the hilum of each lung.
- Describe the divisions of the bronchial tree.
- Outline the blood supply and innervation of the lungs.
- Discuss the mechanics of respiration.

5. The Abdomen

Regions and components of the abdomen

The abdominal cavity is separated from the thoracic cavity by the diaphragm. Because the domes of the diaphragm arch high above the costal margin, the upper part of the abdomen—including the liver, the spleen, the upper poles of the kidneys, and the suprarenal glands—is protected by the bony thoracic cage. The lower part of the abdominal cavity lies within the bony pelvis above the pelvic inlet.

Posteriorly, the vertebral column protects the abdominal contents, but anteriorly and laterally the abdomen is more vulnerable to injury, with only a muscular wall for protection. However, this permits flexibility for respiration and posture.

Over the anterior abdominal wall, a part of the superficial fascia condenses into a strong but thin membranous layer under the fat. This allows the fatty layer of the superficial fascia (Camper's fascia) to move freely during thoracic and abdominal movements (e.g., respiration). This membranous superficial fascia (Scarpa's fascia) fades over the thoracic wall superiorly, and does not continue into the thigh inferiorly. In males it continues into the scrotum and penis as the superficial perineal fascia (Colles') and the superficial fascia of the penis, respectively. In the female the superficial perineal fascia lines the skin of the perineum, and it is split centrally by the presence of the vagina.

The anterolateral abdominal wall is made up of a muscular sheet composed of three muscle layers. These are separated laterally, but they fuse anteriorly to surround the rectus abdominis.

The abdominal cavity contains most of the gastrointestinal tract (stomach, duodenum, and small and large intestines) together with its derivatives (liver and pancreas). Parts of the viscera (e.g., small intestines, transverse colon, and sigmoid colon) are attached to the body wall by a double fold of peritoneum, called a mesentery, while other viscera (e.g., duodenum and the ascending and descending colon) are bound down to the posterior abdominal wall. The kidney, suprarenal glands, and ureters lie in the posterior abdominal wall, behind the peritoneum.

Abdominal pain is a very common presentation, but often difficult to diagnose—knowledge of the embryology and anatomy of the region is crucial to reaching the correct diagnosis (Fig. 5.1).

Surface anatomy and superficial structures

To facilitate description, the abdomen is divided into regions. The simplest method is to divide the abdomen into four quadrants by vertical and horizontal lines through the umbilicus—upper right, upper left, lower right, and lower left quadrants. However, for more accurate description, it can be divided into nine regions by two vertical and two horizontal lines (Fig. 5.2):

- The vertical line on each side corresponds to the midclavicular line, which extends down to the midinguinal point.
- The lower transverse line runs between the two tubercles of the iliac crest (intertubercular plane).
- The upper transverse line lies midway between the pubic symphysis and jugular notch (transpyloric plane), at the tip of the 9th rib.

The linea alba is a midline depression running from the xiphisternum to the pubis. The linea semilunaris is a smooth, curved line, representing the lateral margin of the rectus abdominis.

The inguinal ligament runs from the anterior superior iliac spine to the pubic tubercle. The deep inguinal ring lies at the midinguinal point (halfway between the anterior superior iliac spine and the pubic tubercle).

 The body wall has three muscle layers in the abdomen. These layers fuse centrally to form the rectus sheath.

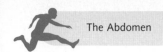

Origin and blood supply of the abdominal viscera			
Part of fetal gut	Organs	Blood supply	Usual site of presentation of abdominal pain
Foregut	Esophagus, stomach, first and second part of the duodenum (to the entrance of the hepatopancreatic duct), liver, pancreas	Celiac artery	Epigastric region
Midgut	Remainder of duodenum, jejunum, ileum, cecum, appendix, ascending colon, right two-thirds of transverse colon	Superior mesenteric artery	Umbilical region
Hindgut	Remainder of the transverse colon, descending colon, sigmoid colon, rectum, and upper half of the anal canal	Inferior mesenteric artery	Suprapubic region

Fig. 5.1 Origin and blood supply of the abdominal viscera.

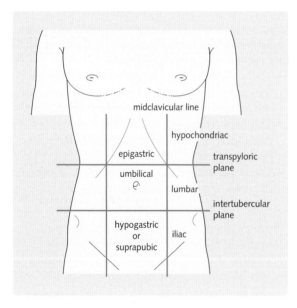

Fig. 5.2 Regions of the abdomen.

from one midclavicular line to the other. The liver lies largely in the right hypochondrium, epigastrium, and extends into the left hypochondrium.

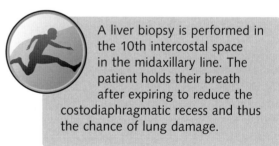

A liver biopsy is performed in the 10th intercostal space in the midaxillary line. The patient holds their breath after expiring to reduce the costodiaphragmatic recess and thus the chance of lung damage.

Fundus of the gallbladder

This lies deep to the intersection of the linea semilunaris with the costal margin in the transpyloric plane. At this point the fundus of the gallbladder lies behind the 9th costal cartilage at the tip of the 9th rib.

Spleen

The spleen lies deep to the 9th, 10th, and 11th ribs in the left hypochondrium at the midaxillary line. It is not palpable unless it is enlarged, at which point the spleen extends inferiorly and anteriorly and can be felt below the costal margin.

Liver

The inferior border extends from the right 10th rib and costal cartilage in the midclavicular line to the left 5th rib in the midclavicular line. The upper border runs between the left and right 5th ribs

Pancreas

The head of the pancreas lies in the C-shaped concavity of the duodenum and with the body at the level of the L2 vertebra. The pancreas continues to the left, curving upwards towards the hilum of the spleen.

Kidneys

The hilum of the left kidney lies in the transpyloric plane, 5 cm from the midline. The upper poles of the kidneys lie on the 11th and 12th ribs posteriorly. The right kidney is 2.5 cm lower than the left due to the presence of the liver, but they both lie roughly opposite the 12th thoracic vertebra and the first two lumbar vertebrae.

Ureters

Each ureter begins at the hilum of the kidney in the transpyloric plane. They run inferiorly over the psoas major muscle in a sagittal plane that intersects the tips of the transverse processes of the lumbar vertebrae (as seen on a pylogram).

The abdominal wall

Skeleton

Fig. 5.3 shows the skeleton of the abdominal and pelvic cavities.

The costal margin and floating ribs (11th and 12th) have been described previously (see Chapter 4).

The coxal (hip) bones articulate with the sacrum at the sacroiliac joint and with each other at the pubic symphysis. Each coxal bone is formed by the ilium, ischium, and pubis.

The iliac bones protect the underlying structures, providing a site for muscle attachment. The upper border—the iliac crest—ends anteriorly at the superior iliac spine (ASIS) and the posteriorly at the posterior superior iliac spine (PSIS) of the iliac crest. The tubercle lies 5–6 cm posterior to the ASIS.

The three sheets of muscle of the anterolateral abdominal wall arise from the iliac crest. The latissimus dorsi, quadratus lumborum, and thoracolumbar fascia are also attached to the crest.

The pectineal line (pectin pubis) lies on the superior surface of the superior ramus of the pubic bone and continues laterally as the arcuate line of

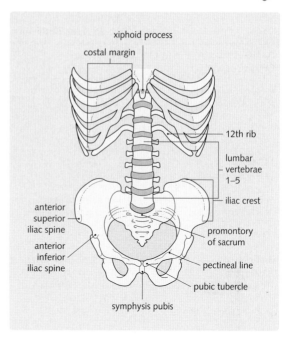

Fig. 5.3 Skeleton of the abdomen and pelvis.

the ilium. Medial to it lie the pubic tubercle and pubic crest.

Thoracolumbar fascia

The lumbar part of this fascia arises in three sheets from:
- Tips of the lumbar and sacral spines (posterior sheet).
- Tips of the lumbar transverse processes (middle sheet).
- The anterior aspect of the lumbar transverse processes (anterior sheet).

The anterior and middle sheets enclose the quadratus lumborum muscle; the middle and posterior sheets enclose the erector spinae muscle. The three sheets fuse laterally and provide attachment for the internal oblique and transversus abdominis muscles. The thoracic part is formed of only a single sheet and is found between the serratus anterior and the erector spinae muscles. This attaches to the thoracic spines and angles of the ribs as far as the first rib.

Muscles of the anterolateral abdominal wall

Fig. 5.4 outlines the muscles of the anterolateral abdominal wall.

83

Muscles of the anterolateral abdominal wall

Name of muscle (nerve supply)	Origin	Insertion	Action
External oblique (T5–T12 spinal nerves)	External surface of ribs 5–12	Becomes aponeurotic and attaches to the xiphoid process, linea alba, pubic crest, pubic tubercle, and anterior half of iliac crest	Fixes and rotates trunk, pulls down ribs in forced expiration
Internal oblique (spinal nerves T6–T12, iliohypogastric and ilioinguinal nerves)	Thoracolumbar fascia anterior two-thirds of iliac crest, lateral half of inguinal ligament	Inferior border of ribs 10–12 and their costal cartilages, pubic crest and pectin pubis via conjoint tendon with transversus	Assists in flexing and rotating trunk; pulls down ribs in forced expiration
Transversus abdominis (spinal nerves T5–T12, iliohypogastric and ilioinguinal nerves)	Internal surface of lower six costal cartilages, thoracolumbar fascia, iliac crest, lateral third of inguinal ligament	Pubic crest, linea alba, symphysis pubis; forms conjoint tendon to pectus pubis with internal oblique	Compresses and supports abdominal contents and flexes external and internal oblique muscles
Rectus abdominis (spinal nerves T6–T12)	Symphysis pubis and pubic crest	Costal cartilages 5–7 and xiphoid process	Compresses abdominal contents and flexes trunk (lumbar vertebrae)

Fig. 5.4 Muscles of the anterolateral abdominal wall.

Rectus sheath

Each rectus abdominis muscle is enclosed in a fibrous sheath formed by the aponeurotic tendons of the three lateral muscles (Fig. 5.5).

The external oblique muscle contributes to the anterior layer of the sheath over its entire extent. Below the costal margin, the internal oblique aponeurosis splits around the muscle, forming the anterior and posterior layers. The aponeurosis of transversus abdominis contributes to the posterior layer. Beneath the posterior layer is transversalis (endoabdominal) fascia and peritoneum.

Approximately midway between the symphysis pubis and the umbilicus, the posterior wall of the sheath becomes deficient, and all of the aponeuroses of the lateral abdominal muscles pass anterior to the rectus muscle. The free lower edge of the aponeurotic posterior wall above this point is called the arcuate line. Below this line and posterior to the rectus muscle is now only transversalis fascia and peritoneum. The inferior

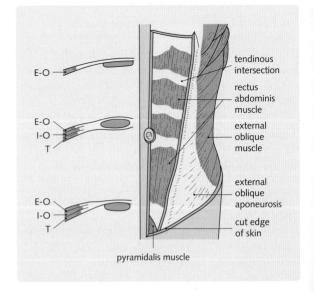

Fig. 5.5 Rectus sheath and rectus abdominis muscle (E-O, external oblique; I-O, internal oblique; T, transversus abdominis).

epigastric artery enters the sheath at the arcuate line, and it runs on the deep surface of rectus abdominis.

The posterior wall of the sheath is also deficient above the costal margin, where the rectus muscle lies directly on the underlying costal cartilages because the transverses abdominis passes posterior to the costal cartilages and the internal oblique attaches to the costal margin.

Nerve and blood supply to the anterolateral abdominal wall

The principal nerves and arteries of the anterolateral abdominal wall are shown in Fig. 5.6.

Venous drainage of the anterolateral abdominal wall

The deep and superficial veins draining the anterolateral body wall include the following:
- The musculophrenic and superior epigastric, which drain to the internal thoracic vein.
- The posterior intercostals and subcostal veins, which empty into the azygos and hemiazygos veins.
- The inferior epigastric and deep circumflex iliac, which drain to the external iliac vein.
- The superficial circumflex iliac and superficial epigastric, which are tributaries of the femoral vein.

Blood may return to the heart via the superficial abdominal veins if the inferior vena cava becomes obstructed.

Inguinal region
Inguinal ligament

The inguinal ligament is the lower free edge of the aponeurosis of the external oblique muscle. It extends from the ASIS to the pubic tubercle, and it gives origin to the internal oblique and transverse abdominis muscles and blends with the fascia lata of the thigh.

Inguinal canal

This is an oblique passage about 6 cm long through the anterolateral body wall, lying above the medial half of the inguinal ligament (Figs. 5.7 and 5.8). It commences at the deep inguinal ring, and it ends at the superficial ring. The canal contains the spermatic cord, the ilioinguinal nerve, and genital branch of the genitofemoral nerve in males, and the round ligament, the ilioinguinal nerve, and genital branch of the genitofemoral nerve in females.

The superficial inguinal ring is a triangular slit in the external oblique aponeurosis, just above and lateral to the pubic tubercle. The contents of the inguinal canal exit through this ring.

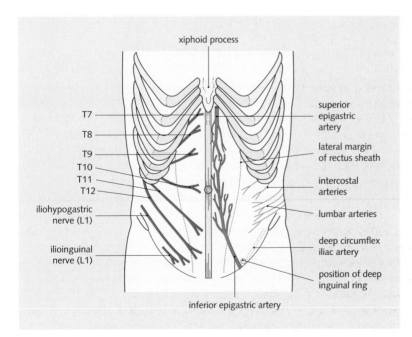

Fig. 5.6 Innervation (left) and arterial supply (right) of the anterolateral abdominal wall.

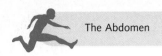

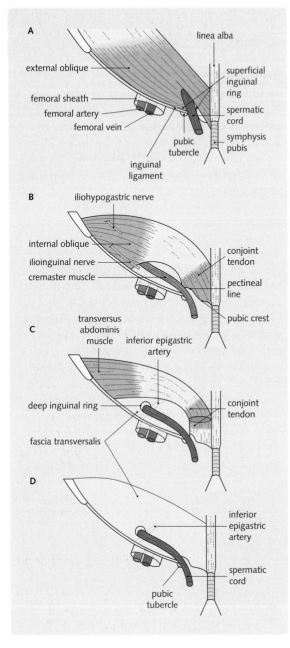

Fig. 5.7 Inguinal canal viewed at different levels.
(A) Superficial inguinal ring in external oblique muscle.
(B, C) Internal oblique and transversus muscles and the
conjoint tendon. (C, D) Deep inguinal ring in fascia
transversalis.

The deep inguinal ring lies at the midinguinal
point and is an opening in the transversalis fascia.
The contents of the spermatic cord and genital
branch of the genitofemoral nerve pass through the
deep inguinal ring.

Composition of the inguinal canal	
Region	**Components**
Anterior wall	External oblique aponeurosis; reinforced laterally by internal oblique
Floor	Lower edge of the inguinal ligament; reinforced medially by the lacunar ligament, which lies between the inguinal ligament and the pectineal line
Roof	Lower edges of the internal oblique and transversus muscles; these muscles arch over the front of the cord laterally, to behind the cord medially, where their joint tendon—the conjoint tendon—is inserted into the pubic crest and pectineal line of the pubic bone
Posterior wall	The strong conjoint tendon medially and the weak transversalis fascia laterally

Fig. 5.8 Composition of the inguinal canal.

The ilioinguinal nerve does not enter the
inguinal canal through the inguinal ring but via
the posterior wall of the canal, emerging from
between the external oblique aponeurosis and the
internal oblique muscle.

Spermatic cord

The structures entering the deep inguinal ring
pick up three coverings from the layers of the
abdominal wall as they pass through the canal to
form the spermatic cord (Fig. 5.9). The spermatic
cord with all of its coverings is not complete until
it emerges from the superficial inguinal ring.

Contents of the spermatic cord comprise:
• The ductus deferens.
• Arteries—the testicular artery (from the
abdominal aorta), the artery to the ductus
deferens (from the inferior vesical artery), and
the cremaster artery to the cremaster muscle.
• Veins—the pampiniform plexus of veins.
• Lymphatics—accompany the veins from the
testis to the lumbar nodes.
• Nerves—the genital branch of the genitofemoral
nerve supplies the cremaster muscle and

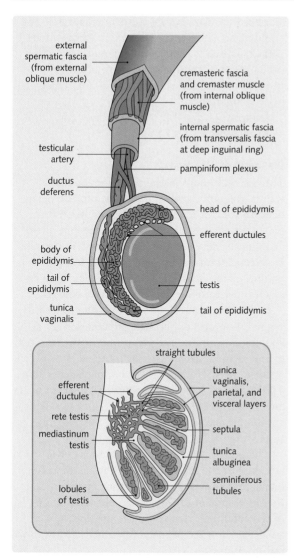

Fig. 5.9 Left testis, epididymis, coverings, and contents of the spermatic cord.

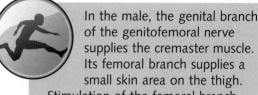

In the male, the genital branch of the genitofemoral nerve supplies the cremaster muscle. Its femoral branch supplies a small skin area on the thigh. Stimulation of the femoral branch causes the cremaster muscle to contract, raising the testis. This is called the cremasteric reflex.

Scrotum

This is a sac-like structure lying below the root of the penis. It contains the testis, the epididymis, and the lower end of the spermatic cord.

Scrotal skin is thin, wrinkled, and pigmented. Beneath this is the superficial fascia, which contains the dartos muscle but no fat. This smooth muscle is attached to the skin and contracts in response to cold, pulling the testes closer to the body and wrinkling the skin. It is supplied by sympathetic nerves. The fascia also forms a septum that separates the testes and is seen externally as the scrotal raphe. The superficial fascia within which the dartos muscle is found is continuous with the superficial perineal (Colles') fascia and the membranous layer of the superficial fascia of the anterior abdominal wall (Scarpa's fascia).

Blood supply, lymphatic drainage, and nerve supply of the scrotum

The posterior scrotal branch of the perineal artery from the internal pudendal, the anterior scrotal branch of the deep external pudendal, and the cremaster artery from the inferior epigastric all supply the scrotum. Scrotal veins accompany the arteries. The lymphatic drainage is via the medial superficial inguinal lymph nodes of the thigh.

The nerve supply to the anterior scrotum is by the ilioinguinal nerve and the genital branch of the genitofemoral anterolaterally. The posterior scrotum is innervated by the posterior scrotal branch of the perineal nerve (medially) and the perineal branch of the posterior femoral cutaneous nerve inferiorly.

sympathetic fibers go to the arteries, and parasympathetic and sympathetic fibers to the ductus deferens.
• The processus vaginalis—may be seen as a fibrous thread representing the obliterated remains of the connection between the abdominal peritoneum and the tunica vaginalis of the testis.

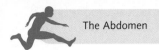

Testis

This oval organ, which produces sperm cells and male hormones, lies in the scrotum (Fig. 5.9). The epididymis is attached to its posterior surface and protrudes laterally. The anterior lateral surface lies free in a serous space between the two layers of the tunica vaginalis—parietal and visceral, a remnant of the fetal processus vaginalis.

Within the visceral tunica vaginalis, the testis has a tough fibrous coat, the tunica albuginea. From its internal surface, numerous septa extend into the gland, dividing it into 200–300 testicular lobules that contain the highly coiled seminiferous tubules. Posteriorly the tubules are joined to straight tubules, which lead to the rete testis, a network of canals. From the rete, sperm are transported by efferent ductules to the head of the epididymis.

Epididymis

This is a long highly coiled tube on the posterior surface of the testis. Its head lies at the upper pole of the testis, where 12–14 efferent ductules join the duct of the epididymis. The body consists of the convoluted duct, which becomes smaller as it passes to the tail and becomes continuous with the ductus deferens.

The epididymis stores sperm and promotes their maturation.

Ductus deferens

This muscular tube conveys sperm from the testis and epididymis to the prostatic urethra. It receives its blood supply from a small artery from the inferior vesical artery. This small artery anastomoses with the testicular artery.

Blood supply of the testis

The testicular artery runs in the spermatic cord, and it supplies the testis and the epididymis. The pampiniform plexus provides venous drainage. In the inguinal canal the plexus merges into four veins, which join to form two right and two left testicular veins before exiting via the deep inguinal ring. The left testicular vein drains into the left renal vein as a single vein, and a right single vein empties into the inferior vena cava. Renal tumors may obstruct the left renal vein, causing dilatation of the veins in the testis, to form a varicocoele.

The testicular artery and its branches are very closely associated with the pampiniform venous plexus. This acts as a countercurrent heat exchanger. For spermatogenesis to occur, the testicular temperature has to be 2–3 °C below body temperature.

Lymphatics drain into the left and right lumbar and pre-aortic nodes.

Descent of the testis

The testis develops in the posterior abdominal wall of the embryo then descends into the pelvis, beneath the peritoneum, until it reaches the presumptive deep inguinal ring by the end of the 3rd month. Between the 7th and the 9th months, it descends into the inguinal canal and then progresses rapidly through the superficial ring to reach the scrotum at around the time of birth.

A diverticulum of peritoneum—the processus vaginalis—proceeds through the anterior abdominal wall into the scrotum, creating the path of the inguinal canal. The testes descend to the scrotum beneath the peritoneum of the processus. The processus is normally obliterated except at its lower end, where it becomes the outer two layers enveloping the testis, the parietal and visceral tunica vaginalis.

The gubernaculum is a ligamentous cord attached to the inferior pole of the testes and the incipient labioscrotal swelling that forms with the development of the testes. The lengthening of the fetal body and the shortening of the gubernaculum are believed to pull the testes down into the scrotum.

The cremaster muscle elevates the testes towards the inguinal canal as part of the cremasteric reflex. This reflex is very active in children, often leading to a misdiagnosis of undescended testes. Failure of the testis to descend, called cryptorchidism, is a serious condition—it may result in impaired fertility, and undescended testes may undergo malignant change.

A hernia is a protrusion of a viscus or part of a viscus through the body wall or into an otherwise abnormal location. Most common hernias are inguinal. Direct inguinal hernias, which are common in adults, push through the posterior wall of the inguinal canal, medial to the inferior epigastric artery and through the superficial inguinal ring. Indirect hernias are seen often in

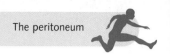

babies, and these result from failure of the processus vaginalis to obliterate. Indirect hernias push through the deep inguinal ring, lateral to the inferior epigastric vessels, and through the inguinal canal; they can descend as far as the scrotum.

The peritoneum

The peritoneum is a serous membrane that consists of mesothelium, a layer of simple squamous epithelial cells. It has two layers continuous with each other:
- The parietal layer lines the internal abdominal wall, the inferior surface of the diaphragm, and the pelvic cavity.
- The visceral layer leaves the abdominal wall and invests the viscera within the abdominal and pelvic cavities.

Embryology
During development, the foregut, midgut, and hindgut are suspended from the posterior abdominal wall by a dorsal mesentery (a mesentery is a double layer of peritoneum that encloses an organ and connects it to the body wall—Fig. 5.10). These organs are known as intraperitoneal.

Some organs lie within the posterior abdominal wall, where they are covered by peritoneum on their anterior surface only (e.g., the kidneys, suprarenal glands, aorta, and superior vena cava). These organs are known as retroperitoneal. Those parts of the gut that lose their mesentery during development (duodenum distal to the entrance of the hepatopancreatic duct, ascending and descending colon) are called secondarily retroperitoneal (see Fig. 5.10).

A ventral mesentery is present in the adult only in the terminal parts of the esophagus and stomach, and the upper part of the duodenum (foregut). It is derived from the ventral mesentery of the foregut, which in this region is called the septum transversum. Growth of the liver into it divides the mesentery into the falciform ligament and the lesser omentum.

Nerve supply of the peritoneum
The parietal peritoneum is supplied segmentally by the nerves supplying the overlying muscles and skin. The peritoneum covering the inferior surface of the diaphragm is supplied by the intercostal

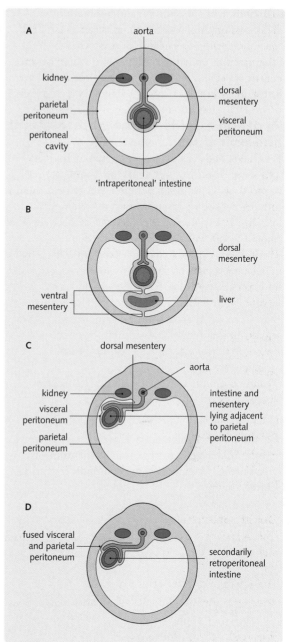

Fig. 5.10 The embryonic dorsal (A) and ventral (B) mesenteries and the formation of the retroperitoneal part of the intestines (C and D). (Adapted from Anatomy as a Basis for Clinical Medicine, by ECB Hall-Craggs. Courtesy of Williams & Wilkins.)

nerves peripherally and by the phrenic nerve centrally. The parietal peritoneum in the pelvis is supplied by the obturator nerve. The visceral peritoneum does not have a somatic innervation, and it is, therefore, insensitive to pain.

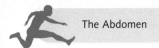

Irritation of the abdominal diaphragm by abdominal pathology is frequently felt as pain in the shoulder region because dermatomes innervated by spinal nerves C3–C5, which also contribute sensory fibers to the phrenic nerve, are found in this region. This is termed "referred pain."

Peritoneal folds of the anterolateral abdominal wall

Peritoneal folds can either be known as folds or ligaments. The term ligaments, as it applies to the peritoneum, describes a double layer of peritoneum running between two structures, e.g., phrenicocolic ligament is a transverse peritoneal fold between the splenic flexure of the colon and the diaphragm.

A fold is a raised area of peritoneum caused by underlying vessels or ducts. Anterolateral peritoneal folds are shown in Fig. 5.11. They include:
- Median umbilical fold—contains the remnant of urachus (median umbilical ligament).
- Medial umbilical folds—contain remnants of the umbilical arteries (medial umbilical ligaments).
- Lateral umbilical folds—contain the inferior epigastric vessels.

The falciform ligament (the peritoneal fold from the anterior abdominal wall between the diaphragm and the umbilicus) contains the ligamentum teres hepatis (the remnant of the left umbilical vein) in its free margin.

Greater and lesser sacs

The space between the parietal and visceral peritoneum is potential, containing a thin film of peritoneal fluid. This is the general peritoneal cavity. In males this peritoneal cavity is completely closed; however, in females the cavity communicates externally via the uterine tubes, uterine cavity, and vagina. The peritoneal cavity is divided into greater and lesser sacs.

The lesser sac (omental bursa) is an enclosed space behind the stomach that communicates with the greater sac, or remaining peritoneal cavity, via the epiploic foramen (of Winslow) beneath the liver. The lesser omentum is formed when the stomach rotates on its vertical and anterior–posterior axes, pulling its ventral mesentery into a coronal plane. The epiploic (omental) foramen is bounded by:
- Superiorly—caudate process of liver.
- Anteriorly—the portal triad of portal vein, proper hepatic artery, and common bile duct in the free edge of the lesser omentum.
- Inferiorly—first part of the duodenum.
- Posteriorly—inferior vena cava.

The greater sac, which is the remainder of the peritoneal cavity, can be divided, descriptively, into compartments by the transverse mesocolon. The supracolic is above, containing the stomach, liver,

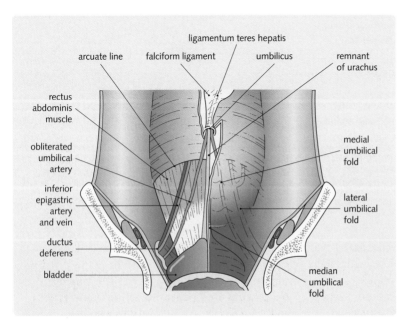

Fig. 5.11 Peritoneal folds of the anterior abdominal wall.

and spleen, with the infracolic compartment below this mesentery, containing the small intestine and ascending and descending colon (Fig. 5.12).

The infracolic compartment is subdivided further by the root of the mesentery (of the small intestine) from the upper right to the lower left of the posterior abdominal wall. The compartment is bounded laterally by the paracolic gutters. The paracolic gutters communicate with the supracolic compartment.

The supracolic compartment is divided into left and right parts by the falciform ligament. Between

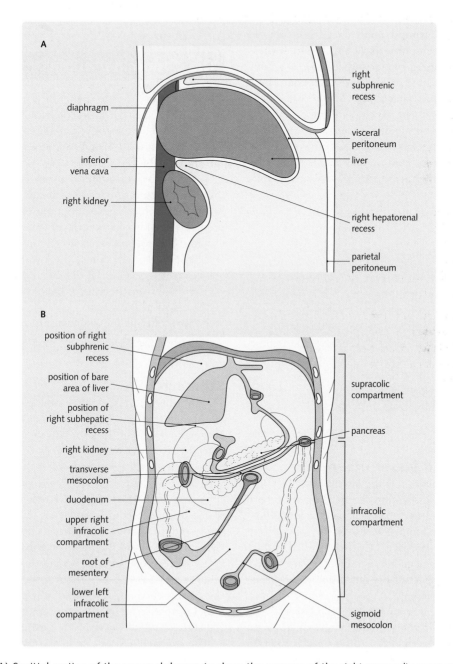

Fig. 5.12 (A) Sagittal section of the upper abdomen to show the recesses of the right supracolic compartment. (B) Posterior abdominal wall showing lines of peritoneal reflection and how the greater sac compartments are divided (liver, stomach, small intestine, cecum, and transverse and sigmoid colons have been removed). ((B) is adapted from Gray's Anatomy, 38th edn., edited by L. H. Bannister et al. Harcourt Brace and Co.)

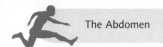

the upper surface of the liver and the diaphragm on either side of the falciform ligament are two spaces, each called a subphrenic recess. Under the liver on the right of the falciform ligament, but above the right kidney, is the right subhepatic recess. The left subhepatic recess has similar boundaries, but it is better known as the lesser sac.

In the pelvic compartment the peritoneum dips over and between pelvic viscera to form pouches that differ between genders. Males have a rectovesical pouch. Females have a vesicouterine and a rectouterine pouch (see Chapter 6).

These recesses and pouches are important since they determine the spread of fluids within the peritoneal cavity, and they are potential sites where infection or fluid may accumulate depending on whether a patient is prone or supine.

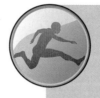
Infection in the subphrenic recess can irritate the diaphragmatic peritoneum, which is innervated by the phrenic nerve. As a result, referred pain is felt in the skin of the shoulder due to a shared C3 and C4 root value between phrenic and cutaneous nerves.

Greater and lesser omenta

The greater omentum is the largest fold of peritoneum. It arises from the greater curvature of the stomach and folds back on itself to attach to the posterior abdominal wall over the pancreas, thus becoming four layers thick. It is filled with fat. The transverse colon and its mesentery are fused to the posterior aspect of the omentum, thus forming a gastrocolic ligament.

The lesser omentum connects the lesser curvature of the stomach and the proximal part of the duodenum to the liver. Although it is a single entity, it can be divided into two parts: a hepatogastric ligament between the liver and stomach and a hepatoduodenal ligament between the liver and duodenum.

The greater omentum is the "policeman" of the abdomen—it can be passively moved to a site of infection and adhere to it, preventing spread.

The abdominal organs

Esophagus

After passing through the diaphragm, the esophagus turns forward and to the left to enter the cardiac part of the stomach. Blood and nerve supply are shown in Fig. 4.27.

Gastroesophageal reflux is a very common problem in young children and in adults. A number of factors have been proposed as preventing reflux of stomach contents into the esophagus. These include:
- The sphincteric action of the lower esophageal muscle.
- The diaphragmatic muscle fibers surrounding the esophageal hiatus.
- Positive intra-abdominal pressure acting on the abdominal esophagus, and reduced intrathoracic pressure.

Stomach

This is a dilated muscular bag joining the esophagus and the duodenum (Fig. 5.13). Its chief function is enzymatic digestion. It is a relatively mobile organ, being fixed only at its ends. The gastroesophageal junction lies just below the level of the T10 vertebra, and the pyloric sphincter (gastroduodenal sphincter) lies at the level of L1 vertebra. The stomach is enclosed in peritoneum that passes from the lesser curvature to the greater curvature. At the lesser curvature the lesser omentum splits into its two layers: one layer passes anteriorly and the other layer passes posteriorly over the stomach. At the greater curvature, the anterior and posterior layers of the lesser omentum are continuous with the anterior double layer of the greater omentum.

The stomach has four parts and two curvatures:
- Cardia—the region surrounding the cardiac orifice from the esophagus.
- Fundus—the dilated superior region under the left dome of the diaphragm and above the plane

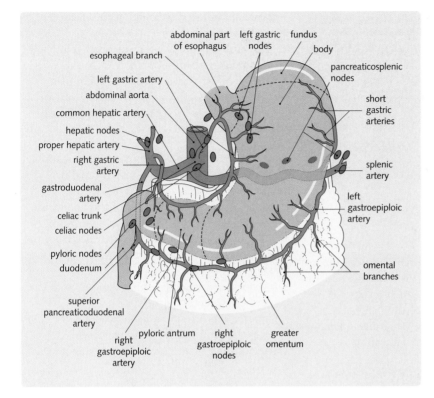

Fig. 5.13 Blood supply and lymphatic drainage of the stomach.

of the cardiac orifice, separated from the esophagus by the cardiac notch; usually filled with gas.
- Body—lies between the fundus and the pyloric antrum.
- Pyloric part—divided into a wide pyloric antrum leading to a narrower pyloric canal. The pyloric orifice, surrounded by the pyloric sphincter, leads to the duodenum.
- Lesser curvature—forms the shorter concave border of the stomach and is marked by the angular incisure, a sharp indentation that marks the boundary between the body and the pyloric part.
- Greater curvature—the longer convex border of the stomach, from which hangs the anterior layer of the greater omentum.

The stomach is capable of considerable dilation and when contracted, its mucosal lining is thrown into gastric folds or rugae. The gastric canal is a longitudinal furrow along the lesser curvature, which forms during swallowing and which carries liquids to the pyloric canal when the stomach is empty. There are outer longitudinal, middle circular, and incomplete inner oblique muscle layers in the stomach wall.

The relations of the stomach comprise:
- Anterior—the anterolateral abdominal wall, left costal margin, diaphragm, and left lobe of the liver.
- Posterior (stomach bed) from superior to inferior—the left dome of the diaphragm, spleen, the left suprarenal gland and the upper pole of the left kidney, splenic artery, pancreas, transverse mesocolon, and colon.

The stomach and esophagus are foregut derivatives, and, therefore, they get their blood supply from the celiac trunk: a branch of the abdominal aorta (see Fig. 5.13).

Lymphatic drainage is illustrated in Fig. 5.13.

The nerve supply to the stomach and esophagus comprises:
- Sympathetic—from the T6–T9 levels of the spinal cord via the greater splanchnic nerve to the celiac plexus to be distributed along arteries. Stimulation decreases secretions and peristalitic activity.
- Parasympathetic—from the anterior and posterior vagal trunks with fibers to and then from the celiac trunk. Stimulation increases secretions and peristaltic activity.

In a sliding hiatal hernia the abdominal esophagus, cardia, and parts of the stomach slide superiorly through the esophageal hiatus. This is due to an age-related weakening of the diaphragmatic right crus, especially when the person is lying down or bending over.

Duodenum

The pyloric portion of the stomach empties into the duodenum. This is the first and shortest part of the small intestine (25 cm), which makes a C-shaped curve around the head of the pancreas. Most of it is secondarily retroperitoneal and firmly attached to the posterior abdominal wall. It is divided into four parts:

- The first part passes posteriorly to the right side of the vertebral column, along the transpyloric plane at the L1 vertebral level.
- The second part passes inferiorly along the right side of the L1–L3 vertebrae and receives the hepatopancreatic ampulla (of Vater), the opening of the bile duct and main pancreatic duct at the level of the L2 vertebra, which empties into the duodenum at the major duodenal papilla.
- The third part crosses the vertebral column at the level of L3 vertebra.
- The fourth part ascends to the level of L2 vertebra and is continuous with the jejunum at the point where the suspensory ligament of Treitz is attached to the duodenum.

The first part of the duodenum is very susceptible to peptic ulcers, which are usually caused by infection with *Helicobacter pylori*.

Fig. 5.14 shows the relations of the duodenum. The duodenum gets its blood supply from:

- Superior pancreaticoduodenal arteries from the gastroduodenal branch of the common hepatic artery.
- Inferior pancreaticoduodenal arteries from the superior mesenteric artery.
- Superior and inferior pancreaticoduodenal veins return blood from the superior mesenteric artery to the superior and inferior mesenteric veins.

Duodenal lymph drains into channels that accompany the superior and inferior pancreaticoduodenal vessels to the celiac and superior mesenteric nodes.

The duodenum is innervated by branches of the vagus nerve and the greater and lesser splanchnic nerves via the celiac plexus.

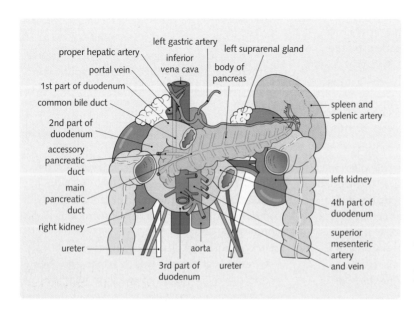

Fig. 5.14 Relations of the duodenum. Note the splenic vein is hidden behind the pancreas and, therefore, not drawn, and the inferior mesenteric vein has been omitted for clarity.

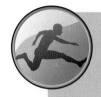

If a duodenal ulcer perforates, gas, digested food, and intestinal bacteria enter the peritoneal cavity. This causes very painful inflammation of the peritoneum (peritonitis).

Jejunum and ileum

The jejunum and ileum lie free in the abdomen. They are attached to the posterior abdominal wall by the mesentery of the small intestine. Their total length is approximately 6–7 m.

Fig. 5.15 outlines the differences between the jejunum and ileum.

The blood supply to the jejunum and ileum is from the jejunal and ileal branches of the superior mesenteric artery. The arteries form a series of anastomotic loops to make arterial arcades. From these arcades, straight arteries (vasa recta) pass to the mesenteric border of the gut. The straight arteries (vasa recta) are end arteries—occlusion may result in infarction.

Lymphatic drainage is to the superior mesenteric nodes.

Parasympathetic fibers from the vagus nerve increase peristalsis and secretion, whereas sympathetic fibers from the lateral horn of T9 and T10 via the greater, lesser, and least splanchnic nerves to the superior mesenteric plexus inhibit peristalsis.

Large intestine

This consists of the cecum, appendix, ascending, transverse, and descending colon, rectum, and upper part of the anal canal.

Cecum and vermiform appendix

The cecum and the vermiform appendix lie in the right iliac fossa, in the lower right quadrant.

The cecum lies free in the abdominal cavity, invested by peritoneum. The ileum enters the cecum obliquely, and partially invaginates into it, forming the ileocecal orifice. Below this entrance, the cecum is a blind pouch. The blood supply to the cecum is from the ileocolic artery, the terminal branch of the superior mesenteric artery.

The vermiform appendix is a worm-shaped blind-ending tube with lymphoid tissue in its wall, and it is usually 6–9 cm long. It opens into the posteromedial wall of the cecum, 2 cm below the ileocecal orifice. The vermiform appendix has its own mesentery, the mesoappendix, and the teniae coli of the colon merge to form a complete layer of longitudinal muscle.

Its blood supply is from the appendicular artery, a branch of the ileocecal or posterior cecal artery. It is an end artery, and any swelling of the vermiform appendix may obstruct the artery, causing necrosis and perforation.

Appendicitis is a common surgical emergency. It usually presents with central abdominal pain, which later spreads to the lower right quadrant. The surface projection of the site of the appendix

Distinguishing characteristics of the jejunum and ileum		
Characteristic	Jejunum	Ileum
Color	Deep red	Paler pink
Wall	Thick and heavy	Thin and light
Vascularity	Greater	Less
Vasa recta	Long	Short
Arcades	A few large loops	Many short loops
Peyer's patches (aggregated lymphoid follicles)	No	Yes—toward the terminal part of the ileum
Plicae circulares (mucosal folds increasing surface area)	More and larger	Less and smaller/absent
Fat in the mesentery	Less	More

Fig. 5.15 Distinguishing characteristics of the jejunum and ileum.

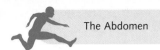

is located at McBurney's point, one third of the way along a line joining the anterior superior iliac spine and the umbilicus.

Colon

Most of the length of the colon has an inner circular muscle layer and an incomplete outer longitudinal muscle layer represented by three bands: the teniae coli. The longitudinal muscle of the vermiform appendix divides into the teniae coli and travel along the length of the colon. In the sigmoid (pelvic) colon the teniae coli are wider, and at the rectosigmoid junction they coalesce to form a complete longitudinal muscle layer.

Haustra (sacculations) are pouches along the length of the colon. These occur because the three teniae coli are shorter than the colon itself, thus shortening the colonic wall.

Pendant-shaped bodies of fat hang from the tenia within a layer of peritoneum. These are the appendices epiploicae. They become larger and more developed along the length of the colon.

Diverticulosis is a disorder in which evaginations of the mucosa of the colon herniates through weak areas of the colon, following nutrient arteries to the submucosa. Such an evagination is called a diverticulum.

Ascending colon

This extends from the ileocolic junction to the right colic (hepatic) flexure. On the lateral side of the ascending colon, there is a deep groove lined with parietal peritoneum, forming the paracolic gutter. The colon is fixed by peritoneum covering its anterior surface and sides that has fused with the parietal peritoneum of the posterior abdominal wall and is thus considered secondarily retroperitoneal.

Transverse colon

This extends from the right colic (hepatic) flexure to the left colic (splenic) flexure, the former being lower due to the presence of the right lobe of the liver. It is completely invested in peritoneum and hangs free on the transverse mesocolon. The left colic flexure is attached to the diaphragm by the phrenicocolic ligament.

Descending colon

This extends from the left colic (splenic) flexure to the left iliac fossa, and like the ascending colon, it is secondarily retroperitoneal. It is fixed to the posterior abdominal wall by the fusion of the peritoneum covering it to the parietal peritoneum. There is a paracolic gutter on its lateral side.

Sigmoid or pelvic colon

This extends from the descending colon to the level of the S3 vertebra, within the true pelvic cavity. It hangs free from the sigmoid mesocolon. The mesocolon is an inverted V-shape, the base of which lies over the sacroiliac joint. One arm runs medially and superiorly along the external iliac vessels, and the other runs inferiorly to the level of the third sacral segment where the rectum begins.

The colon is supplied by the superior mesenteric artery (artery of the midgut) up to the proximal two–thirds of the transverse colon, and the inferior mesenteric artery thereafter (Fig. 5.16).

The branches anastomose near the inner margin of the entire colon, forming an arterial circle, the marginal artery, from which short vessels pass to the gut wall. The weakest part of the marginal artery supply to the colon is between the middle colic and left colic arteries at the splenic flexure, where no anastomosis may occur. This site is thus most prone to ischemia and infarction.

The venous drainage follows the arterial supply to the portal venous system.

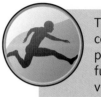 The ascending and descending colons are held onto the posterior abdominal wall by a fusion of the parietal and visceral pleura, i.e., they are secondarily retroperitoneal. The transverse and sigmoid colons are suspended by mesenteries and are mobile.

Fig. 5.16 Colon and its blood supply.

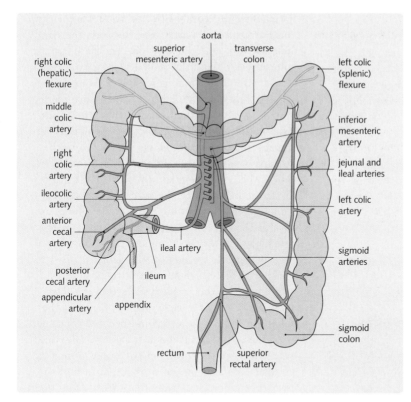

Spleen

The spleen is the largest gland in the body. It removes cellular debris and aged or defective cells from the circulation, and it helps in mounting an immunological response against blood-borne pathogens.

The spleen has a convex diaphragmatic surface that fits into the concavity of the diaphragm. The anterior and superior borders are notched and sharp, but the posterior and inferior borders are rounded.

The spleen is related to the posterior wall of the stomach anteriorly. It is connected to the greater curvature of the stomach by the gastrosplenic ligament and to the posterior abdominal wall at the left kidney by the splenorenal ligament. It is completely enclosed by peritoneum except at the hilum, where the splenic vessels enter and leave.

The splenic artery from the celiac trunk is a tortuous vessel that passes along the superior border of the pancreas, anterior to the left kidney. Between the layers of the splenorenal ligament, the splenic artery divides into five or more branches, which enter the hilum.

The splenic vein joins the inferior mesenteric vein, and this runs posterior to the body and tail of the pancreas to unite with the superior mesenteric vein at the neck of the pancreas to form the hepatic portal vein.

Lymphatic drainage is to the pancreaticosplenic and celiac nodes.

The spleen is the most frequently injured abdominal organ from blows to the left side of the abdominal wall, and it may bleed profusely, resulting in collapse of the patient and shock. An emergency splenectomy may be life saving in these cases. A total splenectomy does not usually produce serious effects, although the risk for infection is increased about 12 times in adults and 50–100 times in children, requiring vaccinations and lifelong treatment with antibiotics.

A perforated gastric ulcer in the posterior stomach wall may erode the splenic artery, as it travels along the superior border of the pancreas, causing it to hemorrhage.

Liver

The liver is a wedge-shaped organ lying in the right upper quadrant and extending into the left. In addition to its many metabolic activities, it stores glycogen and secretes bile. It lies largely under cover of the costal margin, and it is invested by peritoneum except over the bare area on its diaphragmatic surface.

The liver has four lobes (Fig. 5.17). On the inferior surface of the liver, the right lobe is delineated from the left part of the liver by the gallbladder fossa anteriorly and the fossa for the inferior vena cava posteriorly. Between the right lobe and the anatomic left lobe are the quadrate lobe anteriorly and the caudate lobe posteriorly. The anatomic left lobe is separated from the caudate and quadrate lobes by the fissure for the round ligament of the liver and the fissure for the ligamentum venosum, respectively. The porta hepatis is a transverse fissure on the inferior surface between the caudate and quadrate lobes, where the portal vein and proper hepatic artery enter the liver and the hepatic ducts leave. Functionally, the quadrate and caudate lobes are part of the left lobe as they are supplied by the left hepatic artery, left branch of the portal vein, and deliver bile to the left bile duct.

The falciform ligament has a vertical attachment to the anterior surface of the liver. At its superior end, the right and left layers of the falciform ligament diverge and become continuous with the coronary ligament of the liver on either side. The coronary ligament surrounds a roughly circular bare area on the superior surface of the liver. The coronary ligament is formed from anterior (upper) and posterior (lower) reflections of the peritoneum of the diaphragm that are continuous with each other at their right and left edges, thus forming the right and left triangular ligaments (see Fig. 5.17).

The bare area is thus between the upper and lower layers of the coronary ligament. This area is devoid of peritoneum and lies in contact with the diaphragm.

The right and left layers of peritoneum covering the liver meet on the visceral surface of the liver to form the hepatogastric and hepatoduodenal ligaments, both of which constitute the lesser omentum.

Between the caudate and quadrate lobes, the two layers surround the porta hepatis. The inferior vena cava and the gallbladder on the left, the fissures of the ligamentum venosum and ligamentum teres on the right, and the porta hepatis lying transversely between them form an H-shaped pattern. The ligamentum venosum is the remnant of the fetal ductus venosus, which transports blood from the left umbilical vein to the inferior vena cava, short-circuiting the liver.

The porta hepatis contains the right and left branches of the hepatic artery, the hepatic ducts, and the hepatic portal vein (see Fig. 5.17):

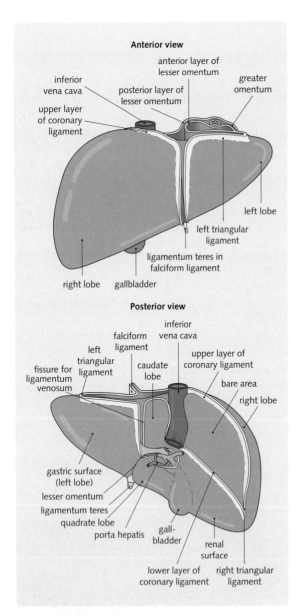

Fig. 5.17 Anterior and posterior views of the liver.

- The common hepatic artery from the celiac trunk divides into the gastroduodenal artery and the proper hepatic artery, which supplies oxygenated blood to the lobes of the liver via its branches, the right and left hepatic arteries. The cystic artery commmonly arises from the right hepatic artery to supply the gallbladder.
- The hepatic portal vein carries more than 70% of the blood to the liver, including all of the nutrients absorbed by the gut.
- The right and left hepatic ducts drain bile into the common hepatic duct. The latter joins the cystic duct to form the common bile duct.

There are also right, intermediate, and left hepatic veins that drain the liver. These do not have an extrahepatic course but drain directly into the inferior vena cava.

Lymphatics drain into the hepatic nodes lying around the porta hepatis and in the lesser omentum. They also drain the gallbladder. These nodes drain into the celiac nodes and from there to the cisterna chyli. Lymphatics of the bare area drain into the posterior mediastinal nodes.

The liver is innervated by parasympathetic fibers from the left and right vagal trunks and sympathetic fibers from the celiac plexus.

Gallbladder and biliary tract

The gallbladder lies in a fossa on the visceral surface of the liver. It has a fundus, a body, and a neck (Fig. 5.18).

The gallbladder stores and concentrates bile secreted by the liver. The bile is released into the duodenum when the gallbladder is stimulated (e.g., after a fatty meal).

The cystic duct drains the gallbladder and joins the common hepatic duct to form the common bile duct. The mucosa lining the neck of the gallbladder and cystic duct is thrown into folds to form a spiral valve, which helps keep the duct open. The bile duct passes through the free margin of the lesser omentum (the hepatoduodenal ligament), behind the first part of the duodenum, to empty into the second part of the duodenum, together with the pancreatic duct, via the hepatopancreatic ampulla (of Vater). The ampulla opens on the summit of a projection on the posteromedial wall of the descending duodenum called the major duodenal papilla. The sphincter of Oddi is a layer of circular muscle surrounding the ampulla. It controls the flow of bile and pancreatic secretions into the duodenum.

Obstruction of the biliary system results in the clinical condition of jaundice (yellow skin).

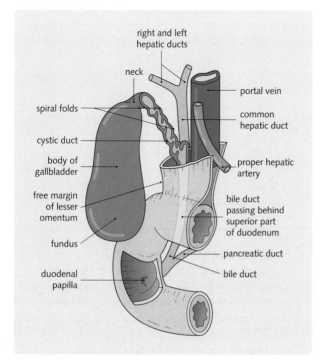

Fig. 5.18 Gallbladder and biliary tract. (Adapted from Anatomy as a Basis for Clinical Medicine, by E C B Hall-Craggs. Courtesy of Williams & Wilkins.)

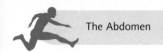

Also, the gallbladder is prone to accumulating concretions called gallstones. These may pass into the duct system, causing severe spasmodic pain (biliary colic).

Blood supply is from the cystic artery, usually a branch of the right hepatic artery. In addition to the cystic veins, veins from the fundus and body drain directly to the visceral surface of the liver.

Pancreas

The pancreas has both exocrine (pancreatic enzymes) and endocrine (glucagon and insulin) functions. It lies transversely behind the peritoneum on the posterior abdominal wall, roughly at the level of the transpyloric plane (see Fig. 5.14). It has a head, neck, body, and tail:

- The head lies in the C-shaped curve of the duodenum, anterior to the inferior vena cava, right renal artery and vein, and left renal vein. The bile duct travels through it. A small projection from the inferior aspect of the head, the uncinate process, extends to the left behind the superior mesenteric artery and vein.
- The neck overlies the superior mesenteric vessels and the portal vein.
- The body crosses the aorta and the L2 vertebra posterior to the omental bursa. The splenic vessels run along the superior margin of this part of the pancreas.
- The tail lies anterior to the left kidney and is accompanied by the splenic vessels and lymphatics between the layers of the lienorenal (splenorenal) ligament, to reach the hilum of the spleen.

The main pancreatic duct opens into the duodenum with the bile duct, via the ampulla of Vater through the major duodenal papilla. The accessory duct opens into the duodenum 2 cm proximal to the major papilla, via the minor duodenal papilla, if present.

The splenic artery, a branch of the celiac trunk, supplies the neck, body, and tail of the pancreas. The superior and inferior pancreaticoduodenal arteries supply the head. The pancreatic veins drain the pancreas via the splenic vein. Lymphatics drain into the celiac and superior mesenteric nodes. The pancreas is innervated by the vagus, the thoracic splanchinic nerves, and fibers from the celiac and superior mesenteric plexus.

Carcinoma of the pancreas has a very poor prognosis, probably because it is silent and asymptomatic for a long time. If the head of the pancreas is involved, the bile duct running through it may become blocked, leading to jaundice. This may alert the clinician sooner.

Vessels of the gut

The foregut, midgut, and hindgut are supplied by the branches of the celiac trunk, the superior mesenteric artery, and the inferior mesenteric artery, respectively.

The celiac trunk arises from the abdominal aorta at the level of T12 vertebra. It gives off the left gastric artery, the common hepatic artery, and the splenic artery (see Fig. 5.13).

The superior mesenteric artery arises from the abdominal aorta at the level of L1 vertebra (transpyloric plane). It gives off the inferior pancreaticoduodenal artery, jejunal and ileal arteries, and the ileocolic, right colic, and middle colic arteries (see Fig. 5.16).

The inferior mesenteric artery arises from the abdominal aorta, opposite L3 vertebra. It gives off the left colic artery, sigmoid arteries, and the superior rectal artery (see Fig. 5.16).

Venous drainage of the gut

Venous blood rich in nutrients from the intestines travels in the hepatic portal system of veins to the liver (Fig. 5.19). The portal vein is formed by the union of the superior mesenteric vein with the splenic vein. The inferior mesenteric vein usually joins the splenic vein.

The portal vein passes posterior to the pancreas and first part of the duodenum to enter the lesser omentum (hepatoduodenal ligament). On reaching the porta hepatis the vein divides into left and right branches supplying the left and right lobes of the liver. From the liver the blood passes to the inferior vena cava via the hepatic veins and then to the heart.

Portal–systemic anastomoses

These are areas where there is a communication between the portal and systemic venous drainage systems. They include the esophagus, the anal canal, the retroperitoneum, and the umbilical region. The most significant of these is the esophagus.

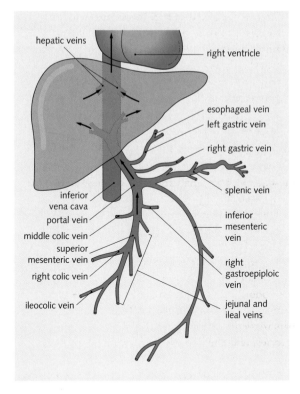

hepatic veins

right ventricle

esophageal vein

left gastric vein

right gastric vein

splenic vein

inferior
vena cava

portal vein

middle colic vein

superior
mesenteric vein

right colic vein

ileocolic vein

inferior
mesenteric
vein

right
gastroepiploic
vein

jejunal and
ileal veins

Fig. 5.19 Hepatic portal venous system.

Portal hypertension caused by liver diseases obstructs portal blood flow and blood is diverted from portal vein tributaries to the systemic veins with which they anastomose. The increased volume through the systemic veins causes them to dilate, forming varices. These may rupture if traumatized, causing severe hemorrhage and even death.

Nerve supply of the gastrointestinal tract: summary

All parts of the gut receive sympathetic nerves that travel with the gut arteries and parasympathetic nerve fibers from the vagus. Sympathetic fibers come from the sympathetic chain and from the celiac, superior mesenteric, and inferior mesenteric plexuses. Parasympathetic fibers for the foregut and midgut enter the abdomen in the left and right vagal trunks, and they are distributed either directly or via the celiac and superior mesenteric plexuses. Parasympathetic supply to the hindgut ascends from the pelvis (S2–S4) in the pelvis parietal peritoneum and the sigmoid mesentery.

Sympathetic fibers inhibit peristalsis and secretion; parasympathetic fibers increase them.

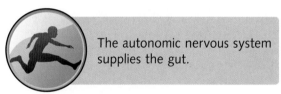

The autonomic nervous system supplies the gut.

Lymphatic drainage of the gut

Lymphatics run with the arteries and end ultimately in lymph nodes lying anterior to the aorta (preaortic nodes) at the roots of its three major branches: the celiac, superior mesenteric, and inferior mesenteric arteries.

Lymph from the mucosa of the gut passes through a number of filters peripherally including:

- Lymphoid follicles, e.g., Peyer's patches.
- The epicolic nodes, which lie directly on the gut.
- The paracolic nodes, which lie between the medial margin of the gut and the root of the mesentery.
- Intermediate or mesocolic nodes that lie along the colic arteries.

All the lymph eventually enters the celiac nodes and from here passes into the cisterna chyli—the origin of the thoracic duct.

Kidneys

The kidneys are retroperitoneal organs that lie on each side of the vertebral column largely under cover of the costal margin on the posterior abdominal wall. The position of the kidneys varies with respiration, but they lie approximately opposite the T12–L3 vertebrae. The right kidney is lower than the left kidney, as it lies below the liver (Fig. 5.20).

The renal hilum is the entrance to the kidney and it is surrounded by a space called the renal sinus, which contains some fat, the renal pelvis—a funnel-shaped expansion at the superior end of the ureter—and vessels and nerves entering and exiting the kidney. In coronal section (see Fig. 5.21), the kidney has a marginal zone called the cortex, which is rich in glomeruli, and a central region called the medulla. The medullary tissue is arranged in the form of inverted pyramids, which

Fig. **5.20** Kidneys and their main anterior relations.

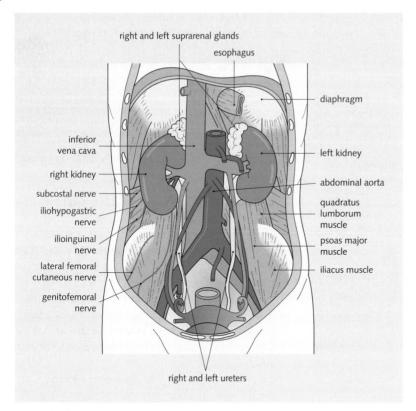

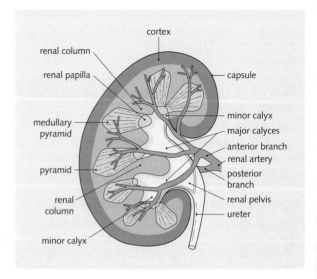

contain straight tubules and collecting ducts. These are separated by renal columns, which contain the ascending and descending loops of Henle. At the tips of the medullary pyramids are renal papillae, which open into the duct system of the kidney:

- Approximately 8 minor calyces.
- 2–3 major calyces.
- Renal pelvis.

Each kidney is surrounded by perirenal fat. The renal fascia encloses the kidney, the suprarenal gland, the perirenal fat, and a fascial septum and separates the kidney from the suprarenal gland. The fascia is firmly attached to the renal vessels and the ureter at the hilum of the kidney. External to the renal fascia is the pararenal fat, retroperitoneal fat of the lumbar region that is mainly posterior to the kidney.

A renal artery supplies each kidney (Fig. 5.21). At the hilum of the kidney the main artery divides into anterior and posterior branches. These are further subdivided into four anterior and one posterior segmental arteries that do not anastomose with the other arteries, making them

Fig. **5.21** Macroscopic structure and arterial supply of the kidney.

102

end arteries. The longer right renal artery passes behind the inferior vena cava. The renal arteries give off an inferior suprarenal artery. Venous drainage is via the segmental veins, which anastomose in variable fashion to form a renal vein. The renal veins join the inferior vena cava at the L2 vertebral level. The left renal vein is longer since it has to pass in front of the aorta and behind the descending superior mesenteric artery to reach the inferior vena cava on its right side. The left renal vein receives the left suprarenal vein, the left gonadal vein, and a branch from the ascending lumbar vein.

A sympathetic nerve supply arises from the aortic, renal, and superior hypogastric plexuses. These carry visceral afferent fibers for pain sensation. A parasympathetic nerve supply is from the vagal trunk but this has an unknown function.

Ureters

The ureters begin at the renal pelvis at the hilum of the kidney. They descend on the psoas muscle behind the peritoneum, and they cross the common iliac artery at its bifurcation at the pelvic brim. They descend on the left wall of the pelvis and turn towards the bladder at the level of the ischial spine.

The ureter narrows in three places:
- At the junction of the ureter and renal pelvis.
- Where it crosses the pelvic brim.
- At its passage into the bladder.

Blood supply is from the renal artery, and variably from the abdominal aorta, the gonadal and vesical arteries, the common and internal iliac arteries, and the middle rectal artery.

The ureter has a sympathetic nerve supply from parts of the aortic plexus and renal plexuses. Parasympathetic fibers come from the pelvic splanchnic nerves. Visceral afferents travel along the sympathetic nerves.

Advanced cases of carcinoma of the cervix may cause renal failure by obstructing the ureters, and they are often fatal.

In the hilum of the kidney, the structures from anterior to posterior are vein, artery, ureter.

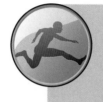

A transplanted kidney is placed in the iliac fossa. The renal vessels are sutured to the external iliac vessels and the ureter is sutured to the bladder.

Suprarenal gland

The suprarenal gland lies on the medial aspect of the superior pole of each kidney, and it is separated from the kidney by the renal fascia. The suprarenal gland consists of a central medulla and a peripheral cortex. The cortex secretes several hormones (e.g., corticosteroids, adrenaline), which are essential for life, while the cells of the medulla are essentially neurons, secreting catecholamines in response to stimulation by presynaptic sympathetic innervation.

The suprarenal gland is supplied by three major arterial sources:
- Six to eight superior suprarenal arteries from the inferior phrenic artery.
- An inferior suprarenal artery from the renal artery.
- One or more suprarenal arteries from the aorta.

The venous drainage of the gland differs slightly on either side. On the right a single suprarenal vein drains into the inferior vena cava directly. On the left a single suprarenal vein drains into the left renal vein. The suprarenal glands are richly innervated by nerves from the celiac plexus and the thoracic splanchnic nerves.

Lymph from the kidneys and the suprarenal glands drains into the lumbar lymph nodes.

The posterior abdominal wall

The posterior abdominal wall offers good protection to the abdominal contents. It is composed of the:
- Bodies of the five lumbar vertebrae and their intervertebral discs.
- Psoas, iliacus, and quadratus lumborum muscles.
- Diaphragm.
- Abdominal fascia.

- Lumbar plexus.
- Fat, nerves, and vessels.

The lumbar vertebrae project with an anterior convexity in the lumbar region (lumbar lordosis). The inferior vena cava lies over the right side and the aorta over the front of the bodies of the vertebrae.

The kidneys and suprarenal glands lie retroperitoneally on either side of the T12–L3 vertebral bodies (Fig. 5.22).

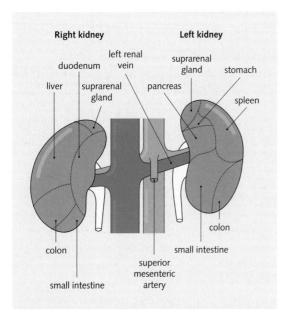

Fig. 5.22 Structures of the posterior abdominal wall.

Muscles of the posterior abdominal wall

These are outlined in Fig. 5.23.

Fascia of the posterior abdominal wall

The muscles of the posterior abdominal wall are covered by thick, strong endoabdominal fascia, which is continuous with the transversalis fascia and provides firm support for the peritoneum and retroperitoneal viscera.

Vessels of the posterior abdominal wall

Abdominal aorta

The abdominal aorta passes through the diaphragm at the level of T12 vertebra. It passes inferiorly on the bodies of the lumbar vertebrae. In front of the body of L4 it divides into the common iliac arteries, which run inferolaterally along the medial border of the psoas muscle as far as the pelvic brim (Fig. 5.24).

Inferior vena cava

This vessel is formed on the right side of the aortic bifurcation, at the level of the L5 vertebra, by the union of the two common iliac veins (see Fig. 4.22). It ascends to the right of the aorta and passes behind the liver to pierce the diaphragm at the level of the T8 vertebra and almost immediately enters the heart. The veins of the posterior abdominal wall are all tributaries of the

Muscles of the posterior abdominal wall			
Name of muscle (nerve supply)	Superior attachment	Inferior attachment	Action
Psoas major (L2–L4)	Transverse process, sides of bodies, and intervertebral discs T12 and L1–L5 vertebrae	Lesser trochanter of femur	With the iliacus, flexes thigh on trunk; laterally flexes the vertebral column
Quadratus lumborum (T12–L4)	Medial half of 12th rib, tips of transverse processes of lower lumbar vertebrae	Iliolumbar ligament, internal lip of iliac crest	Fixes 12th rib during respiration; laterally flexes vertebral column
Iliacus (femoral nerve)	Superior two-thirds of fossa; ala of sacrum	Lesser trochanter of femur; to psoas major tendon	With psoas major, flexes thigh on trunk; stabilizes hip joint

Fig. 5.23 Muscles of the posterior abdominal wall.

inferior vena cava except the left gonadal vein, which empties into the left renal vein.

Nerves of the posterior abdominal wall
Somatic nerves

The upper four lumbar spinal nerves emerge from their intervertebral foramina into the psoas major muscle, which is supplied by branches of L2–L4. Their anterior rami divide and unite to form the lumbar plexus (Fig. 5.25), which mainly provides sensory and motor innervation to the lower limb. However, some branches are motor and sensory to the anterior abdominal wall (e.g., the iliohypogastric nerve), to the medial thigh (e.g., the ilioinguinal and obturator nerves), and to the perineum (e.g., the pudendal nerve). The lumbosacral trunk contains fibers from L4 and L5, which join the sacral plexus.

Autonomic nerves

The autonomic nervous system of the abdomen is composed of the following:

- The vagus nerves and pelvic splanchnic nerves (parasympathetic).

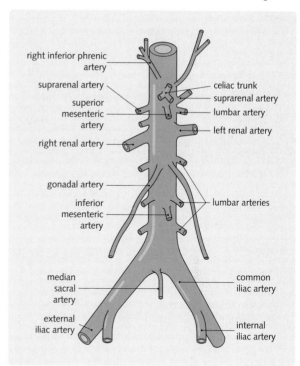

Fig. 5.24 Branches of the abdominal aorta.

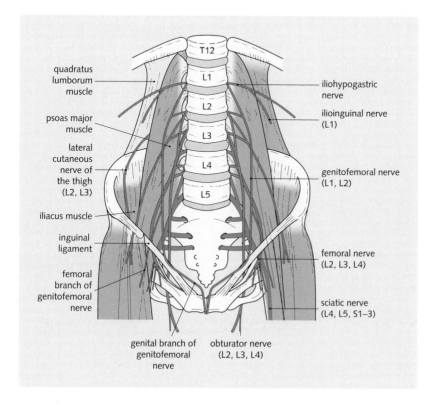

Fig. 5.25 Lumbar plexus and the relationship of the branches to the psoas muscle. The spinal root values of the branches are shown in parentheses. Note the sciatic nerve is not part of the lumbar plexus and is only shown for completeness.

105

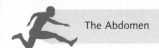

- The lumbar sympathetic trunks, the thoracic splanchnic nerves, and the lumbar splanchnic nerves (sympathetic).

Sympathetic nerves

The lumbar sympathetic trunks are comprised of preganglionic fibers from the lower thoracic trunks and from L1 and L2 nerves (via white rami). These trunks enter the abdomen posterior to the medial arcuate ligaments of the diaphragm. They descend between the medial border of psoas major and the lateral aspect of the bodies of the lumbar vertebrae.

There are usually four lumbar ganglia. These give off gray rami communicantes to all five lumbar nerves, supplying the body wall and lower limb, and visceral branches (lumbar splanchnic nerves from the upper lumbar ganglia) that join the aortic and superior hypogastric plexuses. Preganglion fibers from the third and fourth ganglia join with pre- and postganglionic fibers from the aortic plexus below the bifurcation of the aorta to form the superior hypogastric plexus. The superior hypogastric plexus divides into the right and left hypogastric nerves, which are a loose collection of fibers. These run into the pelvis to join the inferior hypogastric, or pelvic, plexus. These plexuses also contain visceral afferent fibers.

The greater and lesser thoracic splanchnic nerves pierce the crura of the diaphragm to enter the celiac ganglion. The fibers of these splanchnic nerves are preganglionic, and they synapse in the celiac ganglion. The fibers of the least splanchnic nerves synapse in a small aorticorenal ganglion close to the renal arteries.

From the celiac ganglion, postganglionic fibers form a rich network around the aorta and the origin of the celiac trunk, called the celiac plexus. The aortic plexus is similarly dense around the origins of the superior and inferior mesenteric arteries, creating plexuses of the same names. Together, all of the plexuses supply the abdominal viscera via the visceral branches of the aorta. There is also a plexus around the renal artery with fibers going to the kidney.

Pregangion fibers from the lesser splanchnic nerve and also from the celiac plexus innervate the suprarenal gland by synapsing on cells in the suprarenal medulla. The stimulation of these cells causes the release of adrenaline, so they act as postsynaptic sympathetic neurons.

Functions of the sympathetic nerves include vasomotor, motor to the sphincters, inhibition of peristalsis, and as a pathway for sensory fibers from all of the abdominal viscera.

Parasympathetic nerves

The vagal trunks enter the abdomen on the surface of the esophagus. Branches to the celiac plexus supply the gut as far as the distal end of the transverse colon. Branches to the renal plexus innervate the kidneys. The distal part of the transverse colon and the descending and sigmoid colons receive parasympathetic innervation from the pelvic splanchnic nerves.

Functions of the parasympathetic nerves increase peristaltic activity and are secretomotor to the gut and glands.

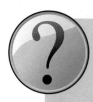

- Outline the boundaries of the abdominal cavity, both skeletal and muscular.
- Discuss two methods for dividing the abdomen into regions.
- Describe the surface projections of four abdominal organs.
- What is the rectus sheath?
- What are the boundaries and contents of the inguinal canal?
- List the contents of the spermatic cord.
- Describe the various ligaments and folds created by the peritoneum in the abdomen.
- Describe how the greater sac is divided into recesses/pouches. Why are these important?
- Define the term omental bursa, how it is formed, and its anatomic relationships.
- List the anatomic relationships of the stomach.
- Outline the differences between the jejunum and ileum.
- Describe the anatomy of the colon.
- Describe the ligaments on the liver formed by peritoneal reflections.
- Describe the anatomic relationships of the pancreas.
- Discuss the blood supply of the gastrointestinal tract.
- Describe the nerve supply of the gastrointestinal tract.
- Describe the lymphatic drainage of the abdominal cavity.
- Name the paired and unpaired branches of the abdominal aorta and the approximate vertebral level at which they arise.
- Describe the formation of the portal vein.
- Define portal–systemic anastomoses, their location, and significance.
- List the branches of the lumbar plexus and identify their spinal nerve roots.
- Describe the anatomy of the kidney.
- Describe the blood supply to the suprarenal glands.

6. The Pelvis and Perineum

Regions and components of the pelvis

The pelvis lies below and behind the abdomen, and it is where the trunk communicates with the lower limbs. It is enclosed by bony, muscular, and ligamentous walls.

The bony pelvis is formed by the two hip (coxal) bones, the sacrum, and coccyx. It has an upper part, the greater pelvis, which contains the inferior abdominal viscera and is flanked by the wings or ala of the iliac bones, and a lower part, the lesser pelvis, which surrounds the pelvic cavity and protects the pelvic viscera. The greater and lesser pelves meet at the pelvic brim (Fig. 6.1) or inlet, which can be defined by its boundaries (see Fig. 6.3).

The pelvic cavity is continuous with the abdominal cavity, and it is, therefore, lined by the peritoneum of the greater peritoneal sac. The peritoneum passes down into the pelvis to cover partially the terminal portions of the gastrointestinal tract, the bladder, and the internal reproductive organs of the female.

The contents of the lesser or true pelvis include:
- The rectum and parts of the sigmoid colon.
- The ureters and bladder.
- The ovaries, uterine tubes, uterus, and vagina in females.
- The ductus deferens, seminal vesicles, and prostate in males.
- The lumbosacral trunk, obturator nerve, sympathetic trunks, sacral plexus, and pelvic plexus.
- The external and internal iliac arteries and their branches, gonadal arteries, and superior rectal arteries.

Surface anatomy and superficial structures

Bony landmarks
The iliac crest can be felt along its entire length. The anterior superior iliac spine is at the anterior border of the iliac crest and lies in the fold of the groin superiorly. The posterior superior iliac spine is at the posterior end of the iliac crest. It lies under a skin dimple at the level of S2 vertebra.

The pubic tubercles can be felt on the upper border of the pubic bone, on either side of the symphysis pubis. The symphysis pubis joins the two pubic bones anteriorly. The pubic crest is a ridge of bone on the superior surface of the pubic bone, medial to the pubic tubercle. The pubic arch is formed by the ischiopubic rami on either side and runs to the ischial tuberosities. The subpubic angle is where these rami meet at the pubic symphysis

The spinous processes of the sacrum fuse to form the median sacral crest. The crest can be felt beneath the skin in the gluteal cleft. The sacral hiatus is found at the lower end of the sacrum, about 5 cm above the coccyx. This leads to the sacral canal. The coccyx may be palpated about 2.5 cm behind the anus.

Viscera
The bladder is a pelvic organ in the adult, but when full it may be palpated through the anterior abdominal wall just superior to the pubic symphysis.

The nonpregnant uterus is not usually palpable. In pregnancy the fundus of the uterus may be palpated from about week 12. At term, the fundus is usually at the level of the xiphoid process.

In a rectal examination of a male the following structures can be palpated:
- The bulb of the penis (anteriorly).
- The membranous urethra (anteriorly).
- The prostate and seminal vesicles (anteriorly).
- The sacrum (posteriorly).
- The coccyx (posteriorly).
- The ischial spines and tuberosities (posterolaterally).

In the female the structures palpated posteriorly are the same as in the male. Anterior structures palpated are:
- The body of the uterus.
- The cervix.

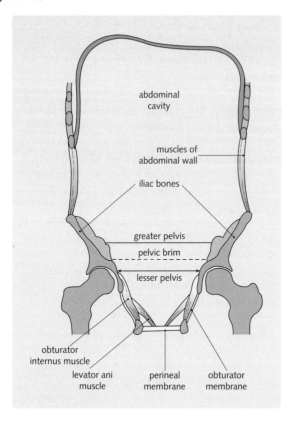

Fig. 6.1 Outline of the pelvic cavity.

In a vaginal examination the following are palpated:
- The lips of the external os.
- The base of bladder and urethra (anteriorly).
- Enlarged uterine tubes (laterally).
- The ovaries (laterally).
- The rectouterine pouch of Douglas (posteriorly).

The bony pelvis and pelvic wall

Bony pelvis
The bony pelvis is formed by the two hip (coxal) bones, the sacrum, and the coccyx (Fig. 6.2). The hip bones meet anteriorly at the pubic symphysis; posteriorly they articulate with the sacrum at the sacroiliac joints. The bony pelvis thus forms a basin that protects the pelvic contents sitting within it.

The pelvis is divided into the greater pelvis (false pelvis), which lies above the pelvic brim (pelvic inlet), and the lesser pelvis (true pelvis),

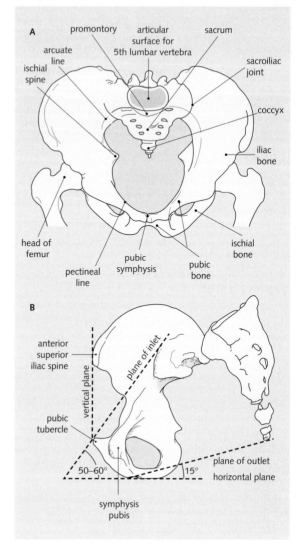

Fig. 6.2 (A) Pelvic girdle. (B) Pelvic inlet and outlet in a normal anatomic position.

which lies between the pelvic inlet and pelvic outlet (Fig. 6.3). The pelvic inlet lies at about 45 degrees to the pelvic outlet.

Sacrum
The sacrum consists of the fused five sacral vertebrae (Fig. 6.4). There are anterior and posterior sacral foramina for passage of the anterior and posterior rami of the sacral spinal nerves. The median sacral crest represents the fused spinal processes of the sacral vertebrae.

The sacrum articulates with the hip bone via its articular surface at the sacroiliac joints.

Fig. 6.3 Boundaries of the pelvic apertures.

Boundaries of the pelvic aperture	
Pelvic inlet	**Pelvic outlet**
Superior border of the pubic symphysis	Inferior margin of the pubic symphysis
Posterior border of the pubic crest	Ischiopubic ramus and the ischial tuberosity
Pectineal line	Ischial tuberosity
Arcuate line of the ilium	Sacrobulbous ligaments
Anterior border of the ala of the sacrum	Tip of the coccyx
Sacral promontory	

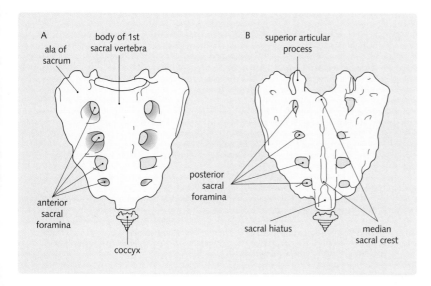

Fig. 6.4 (A) Anterior and (B) posterior views of the sacrum.

Hip bone

This is also called the coxal bone and is formed by the fusion of the ilium, the ischium, and the pubic bone shortly after puberty (Fig. 6.5).

Ilium

The iliac fossa gives rise to the iliacus muscle, and the articular surface contributes to the sacroiliac joint. The iliac crest, and the anterior superior and posterior superior iliac spines define its boundary superiorly. There are also anterior inferior and posterior inferior iliac spines (see Fig. 6.5), which serve as muscle attachments.

The ilium contributes to the formation of the acetabulum and the bony margin of the greater sciatic notch.

Pubis and ischium

The pubic bones articulate in the midline at the pubic symphysis (see Fig. 6.5). On the upper surface of the body are the pubic crest and pubic tubercle. Each pubic bone has a superior and inferior ramus. The superior ramus forms the superior border of the obturator foramen. The inferior ramus unites the pubis with the ischial bone to form the ischiopubic ramus, which ends at the ischial tuberosity, above which lies the body of the ischium.

The posterior border of the ischium contributes to the formation of the greater and lesser sciatic notches. The two notches are separated by the ischial spine. The sacrotuberous and sacrospinous ligaments transform the notches into the greater and lesser sciatic foramina.

> The three bones of the hip all contribute to the formation of the acetabulum.

The position of the pelvis

The pelvis in a standing individual is tilted, such that the anterior superior iliac spine and the superior border of the pubic symphysis lie in the same vertical plane. A horizontal plane runs through the superior border of the pubic symphysis and coccyx.

Male and female pelves

The male and female pelves may show a great deal of sexual dimorphism (Fig. 6.6).

The largest diameter of the pelvic inlet is the transverse diameter (Fig. 6.7), while the largest diameter of the pelvic outlet is the anteroposterior diameter. As the fetal head enters the pelvic inlet,

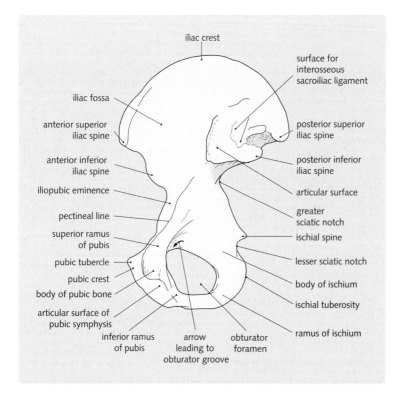

Fig. 6.5 Medial view of the hip bone.

Differences between the male and female pelves		
	Male	Female
Acetabulum	Large	Small
Build	Robust	Light
Inferior pelvic aperture (pelvic outlet)	Relatively small	Relatively large
Obturator foramen	Round	Oval
Pubic arch	Narrow	Wide
Superior pelvic aperture (pelvic inlet)	Usually heart-shaped	Usually oval or rounded

Fig. 6.6 Differences between the male and female pelves.

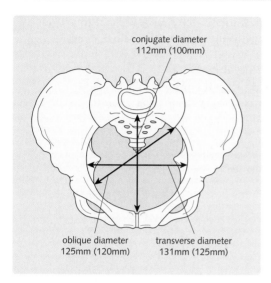

Fig. 6.7 Female pelvic inlet and its average diameters (male average diameters).

it is flexed at the neck to reduce its maximum diameter and as it descends through the birth canal the head rotates externally through 90 degrees, so that it can be accommodated by the wider transverse diameter of the pelvis. When the head reaches the pelvic outlet, it rotates 90 degrees internally so that its maximum diameter lies anteroposteriorly at the pelvic outlet. Failure of this rotation leads to arrest in the delivery, and instrumental assistance (e.g., forceps) or a cesarean section may be required.

Pelvic joints and ligaments
Pubic symphysis
This is a secondary cartilaginous joint between the two pubic bones (see Fig. 6.5). It is usually immobile, except in women in the latter half of pregnancy, and it is reinforced by the superior pubic ligament and the arcuate pubic ligament.

Sacroiliac joint
This is a synovial joint, but because it is a compound joint, it allows only minimal movement. It is strengthened posteriorly by a syndesmosis between the sacrum and the ilium and by strong interosseous ligaments. Weaker anterior and posterior ligaments also stabilize the joint. The joint transmits the weight to the ilia and then to the femurs.

Accessory ligaments to the sacroiliac joints are the sacrotuberous and sacrospinous ligaments (see

Fig. 6.2). The sacrotuberous ligament is flat and wide, running from the ischial tuberosity laterally to the sides of the inferior sacrum and coccyx medially. The sacrospinous ligament is attached to the ischial spines laterally and the sides of the sacrum and coccyx medially. This ligament converts the greater sciatic notch into the greater sciatic foramen and, together with the sacrotuberous ligament, converts the lesser sciatic notch into the lesser sciatic foramen. Posterior rotation of the sacrum and coccyx is prevented by these ligaments.

During the latter half of pregnancy a hormone (relaxin) causes the pelvic joints and ligaments to relax. As a result greater movements occur in the pelvis at the sacroiliac joints and pubic symphysis.

Pelvic wall and floor
The side wall of the pelvis is composed of the coxal bones, lined by the obturator internus muscle and overlying obturator fascia (Fig. 6.8). The posterior wall is formed by the sacrum, the coccyx, and the piriformis muscle as it passes into the greater sciatic foramen.

The pelvic floor is a funnel-shaped layer of muscle, called the pelvic diaphragm, that encloses the terminal parts of the rectum, prostate, and urethra in the male, and the vagina and urethra in the female (Fig. 6.9).

The pelvic diaphragm is composed of the levator ani and the coccygeus muscles. The levator ani has three parts—the pubococcygeus, the iliococcygeus, and the puborectalis. The pubococcygeus portion arises from the posterior surface of the superior ramus of the pubic bone and the anterior arcus tendineous. The iliococcygeus arises from the arcus tendineous posterior to the pubococcygeus and is a very thin layer. The puborectalis can be seen only on the external surface of the levator and consists of the most medial and thick muscle fibers that unite with those of the opposite muscle to form a muscular sling around the anorectal junction. An important function of the levator ani is to increase intraabdominal pressure, which is an important action in forced expiration, coughing, sneezing, vomiting, urinating, defacating, the maintenance of fecal continence, and support of the uterus.

Fig. 6.10 outlines the muscles of the pelvic wall and floor. The arcus tendineus is a thickening of

the obturator internus fascia and runs from the body of the pubis to the ischial spine.

Perineal body

The perineal body is a midline knot of fibromuscular tissue lying posterior to the prostate

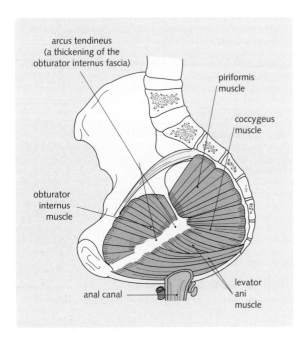

Fig. 6.8 Pelvic wall and its muscles.

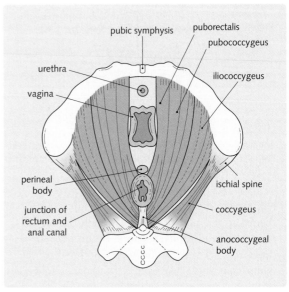

Fig. 6.9 Pelvic floor viewed from below.

Muscles of the pelvic wall and floor			
Name of muscle (nerve supply)	Origin	Insertion	Action
Coccygeus (4th and and 5th sacral nerves)	Ischial spine	Inferior aspect of sacrum and coccyx	Forms part of pelvic diaphragm that supports pelvic viscera, flexes coccyx
Levator ani (pudendal nerve, 4th sacral nerve (pubococcygeus, iliococcygeus, puborectalis)	Ischial spine Body of pubis Fascia of obturator internus	Perineal body Anococcygeal body Walls of prostate, vagina, rectum, and anal canal	Supports pelvic viscera; sphincter to anorectal junction Resists increased abdominal pressure (e.g., defecation, parturition)
Piriformis (first and second sacral nerves)	Pelvic surfaces of 2nd–4th sacral segments, greater sciatic notch, and sacrotuberous ligament	Greater trochanter of femur	Abducts femur at hip and keeps head of femur in acetabulum
Obturator internus (nerve to obturator internus: L5, S1, S2)	Obturator membrane and pelvic surface of ilium and ischium	Greater trochanter of femur	Rotates femur laterally at hip and keeps head of femur in acetabulum

Fig. 6.10 Muscles of the pelvic wall and floor.

or vagina. Parts of the levator ani, the bulbospongiosus muscle, the external sphincter of the anal canal, and the superficial and deep transverse perineal muscles are attached to it. The position and insertion of these muscles into the perineal body provides an essential supporting role for pelvic and perineal structures.

Stretching or tearing of these muscles to the perineal body during childbirth removes the support of the pelvic floor and may result in prolapse of the bladder, vagina, and uterus.

Anococcygeal body/ligament

The anococcygeal ligament or body is a fibrous midline raphe running from the anal canal to the tip of the coccyx, and into which the levator ani muscle inserts. The raphe also separates the two ischiorectal fossae behind the anal canal. The two ischiorectal fossae are continuous below this ligament.

Pelvic fascia

Pelvic fascia is connective tissue having two components:

- A parietal layer that occupies the space between the parietal peritoneum and the muscular walls of the pelvis and is continuous with the endoabdominal fascia superiorly.
- A visceral layer of variable thickness that lies between the visceral peritoneum and the organs that it covers.

The spinal nerves lie external to the fascia and the vessels lie internal to it. The sacral plexus lies between the fascia and the piriformis muscles.

These two layers of the pelvic fascia are continuous with each other where the organs penetrate the pelvic floor and form thickened, tendinous arches running from the pubic bone to the sacrum on either side. The anteriormost portion of this arch is called the puboprostatic and pubovesical ligament in the male and female, respectively. These fibromuscular bands, on either side of the median plane, run from the pubic bone to the bladder neck in the female and to the prostate in the male. They immobilize the bladder neck and support the bladder. Between the ligaments the deep dorsal vein of the penis (or clitoris) passes.

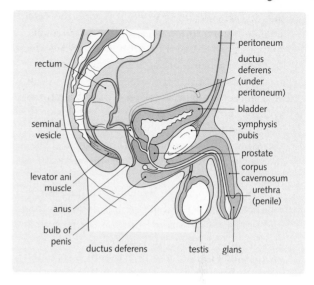

Fig. 6.11 A section through the male pelvis, illustrating the rectum and rectovesical pouch.

Pelvic peritoneum: folds and pouches

In the male, the peritoneum from the pelvic brim lines the pelvic wall and cavity inferiorly. From the anterior abdominal wall the peritoneum is reflected onto the superior surface of the bladder. The bladder lies relatively free in the subperitoneal fatty tissue except at its neck, and this allows it to ascend into the anterior abdominal wall of the greater pelvis as it fills. Behind the bladder, the peritoneum descends before ascending onto the rectum then sacrum. The dip between the bladder and the rectum forms the rectovesical pouch (Fig. 6.11).

In the female the peritoneum reflects from the surface of the bladder onto the anterior wall of the uterus, forming a shallow vesicouterine pouch. After covering the fundus of the uterus, it descends over the posterior wall of the uterus and upper vagina, then ascends to cover the rectum then sacrum. This reflection forms the rectouterine pouch of Douglas (see Fig. 6.16).

The pelvic contents

Pelvic organs
Rectum

The rectum commences as a continuation of the sigmoid colon (where the sigmoid mesocolon ends) at the level of the S3 vertebra and follows the

115

curve of the sacrum to where it pierces the pelvic floor to become the anal canal. The puborectalis muscle maintains an 80 degree anorectal flexure at this point, which is an important mechanism in fecal continence.

The rectum has three lateral curves, and there are also three transverse folds due to folds of the mucosa and muscular submucosa. The folds correspond to the positions of the curves. The lowest part of the rectum dilates as the rectal ampulla.

The rectum has no mesentery. Peritoneum covers the upper third of the rectum at the front and sides, and the middle third of the rectum at the front. The lower third lies below the level of the peritoneum, and the peritoneum is reflected onto the bladder or vagina to form the rectovesical or rectouterine pouch (of Douglas). These pouches are the lowest parts of the peritoneal cavity, and they can be filled with small bowel and the sigmoid colon (see Fig. 6.11). The teniae of the sigmoid colon spread out to give the rectum a complete layer of longitudinal muscle and, therefore, no haustra (sacculations) are present. The rectum also lacks appendices epiplociae.

Posteriorly the rectum is related to the sacrum, coccyx, and pelvic floor.

Vessels and nerves of the rectum

Blood supply is from the superior, middle, and inferior rectal arteries. The superior rectal artery is a continuation of the inferior mesenteric artery. The others are discussed in the section describing the blood supply to the pelvis.

The rectal plexus of veins drains into the inferior mesenteric vein (portal system of veins). The rectal plexus is also drained by the middle and inferior rectal veins. These are systemic veins, i.e., there is portal–systemic anastomosis in the rectum. The longitudinal venous channels of the rectum may dilate to form hemorrhoids. Internal hemorrhoids are prolapses of the rectal mucosa containing the dilated veins. Although they are not painful, they can strangulate or ulcerate. External hemorrhoids occur in the external venous plexus under the skin of the anal canal. These are painful, and unlike internal hemorrhoids, are caused by portal hypertension, as well as pregnancy and constipation.

The nerve supply of the rectum consists of:

- Sympathetic—lumbar sympathetic trunk and hypogastric plexus.
- Parasympathetic—pelvic splanchnic nerves, which are motor to the rectal muscles.

The rectum is distinguished from the sigmoid colon by the lack of a mesentery.

In Hirschsprung's disease, autonomic ganglia are absent from the wall of the sigmoid colon and rectum. This part of the bowel is collapsed, and this leads to bowel obstruction, inflammation, constipation, and vomiting.

Lymphatics from the superior half of the rectum accompany branches of the superior rectal arteries and eventually drain to the lumbar and the inferior mesenteric nodes. Lymphatics from the inferior half of the rectum drain along the middle rectal vessels to the internal iliac nodes.

Ureters in the pelvis

The ureters cross the pelvic brim at the bifurcation of the common iliac vessels (Fig. 6.12). They

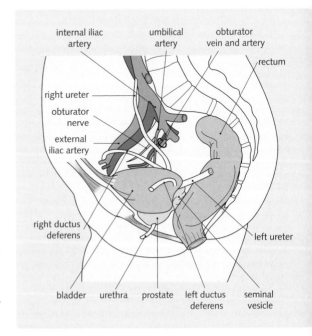

Fig. 6.12 Course of the ureters in the pelvis of the male.

descend on the lateral wall into the lesser pelvis towards the ischial spines and cross the internal iliac vessels. At the pelvic floor they run forward to enter the base of the bladder. In males, the ductus deferens crosses the ureter superiorly; in females, the uterine artery crosses the ureter.

The ureter may be damaged in hysterectomy (removal of the uterus) when it may be tied along with the uterine artery.

> To recall that the female ureter is crossed by the uterine artery superiorly remember 'bridge over troubled water.'

Bladder

The undistended bladder is shaped like the prow of a ship (see Figs. 6.12 and 6.13). The apex points towards the pubic symphysis and the median umbilical ligament (urachus) is attached to it and extends superiorly from it onto the anterior abdominal wall.

The base or posterior surface is triangular. In males, the base lies largely below the rectovesical pouch and it is not covered by peritoneum. The

ductus deferens and the seminal vesicles are located on the surface of the base, and the ureter enters the bladder through its superolateral surface. In females, the base is directly related and attached to the vaginal wall and the upper part of the cervix by connective tissue.

Two inferolateral surfaces become continuous with each other at the retropubic space.

The superior and part of the posterior surface of the bladder is covered by visceral peritoneum. A smooth muscle layer, the detrusor muscle, is an interlacing network of nonstriated muscle fibers, and this gives the bladder a trabeculated appearance. The detrusor muscle has a parasympathetic nerve supply from the vesical plexus, a subdivision of the pelvic plexus. A separate layer of smooth muscle exists at the ureterovesical junction to prevent reflux of urine. The muscle at the neck of the bladder differs from the detrusor muscle histologically, and it has a mainly sympathetic nerve supply. An inner mucosal layer of transitional epithelium lines the bladder.

The urethra leaves the neck of the bladder. In the neck, in males, the muscle is arranged in a circular fashion. This constitutes the internal urethral sphincter, which prevents retrograde ejaculation (sperm entering the bladder). In females the muscle is arranged longitudinally and this sphincter is lacking.

Internal surface of the bladder

When the bladder is empty, the mucosa, which is only loosely attached to the muscle layer, is thick and folded. As the bladder fills, the mucosa becomes thinner and smoother.

The trigone is a triangular area lying between the urethral orifice and the two ureteric orifices. Here the mucosa is adherent to the muscle layer and is always smooth. The interureteric fold or crest, formed by a continuation of the ureteric muscle into the bladder wall, connects the two ureteric orifices.

The ureters pierce the mucosa obliquely, and the valve-like flap of mucosa produced is important in preventing reflux of urine when intravesical pressure increases. The ureteric orifices are closed by this pressure and opened by peristaltic activity. Abnormal entrance of the ureters into the bladder may lead to reflux of urine up into the ureters as far as the pelves and calyces

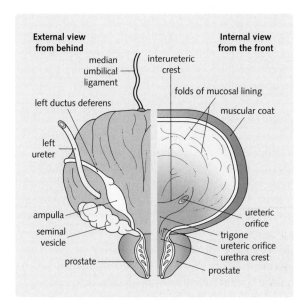

Fig. 6.13 Base of the bladder and related structures in the male.

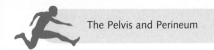

of the kidney. This is a common problem in children and it may result in hypertension and renal failure.

Vessels and nerves of the bladder

Blood supply is from the superior and inferior vesical arteries, with minor contributions from the obturator, uterine, inferior gluteal, and vaginal arteries.

In males, veins on the inferolateral sides of the bladder form a complicated plexus, which drains into the internal iliac veins.

The nerve supply comprises:

- Parasympathetic (motor)—pelvic splanchnic nerves.
- Sympathetic—the superior hypogastric and pelvic plexuses.

Visceral afferents carry pain sensation and an awareness of distention via both parasympathetic and sympathetic pathways.

In males and females a distended bladder rises above the symphysis pubis and lifts the peritoneum away from the anterior abdominal wall. A needle can be inserted above the symphysis pubis to drain the bladder (suprapubic cystostomy) without entering the peritoneal cavity.

The male urethra

The male urethra is 20 cm long, commencing at the bladder neck and terminating at the external urethral orifice (Fig. 6.14). It has three parts:

- The prostatic urethra is the most distensible part, which descends through the prostate gland. It has an elevated central region on its posterior wall, the urethral crest. The rounded eminence on the crest is the seminal colliculus with a slit-like orifice leading to the prostatic utricle. The orifices of the ejaculatory ducts open into the prostatic utricle.
- The membranous urethra lies between the apex of the prostate and the bulb of the penis. It is surrounded by the sphincter urethrae. It penetrates the perineal membrane to become

the spongy urethra. The bulbourethral glands lie on either side of it.

- The spongy urethra passes through the bulb, corpus spongiosum, and glans of the penis. Immediately before the external urethral orifice, the urethra expands to form the navicular fossa.

Numerous urethral glands open throughout the course of the urethra.

The female urethra

The female urethra is only 4 cm long. It runs from the bladder neck through the pelvic floor, where it becomes surrounded by the sphincter urethrae. It then pierces the perineal membrane, to open into the vestibule of the vulva anterior to the vaginal opening.

The female urethra, being shorter than that of the male, is more prone to bacterial urinary tract infections.

Male reproductive organs in the pelvis

Ductus deferens

The ductus deferens passes from the epididymis to the pelvic cavity via the inguinal canal. At the deep inguinal ring it hooks around the inferior epigastric artery, crossing the external iliac vessels to enter the pelvic cavity. It crosses the obturator neurovascular bundle and the ureter to reach the base of the bladder (see Fig. 6.13). The terminal part dilates, forming the ampulla, and it joins the duct of the seminal vesicle to form the ejaculatory duct, which opens into the prostatic urethra on the seminal colliculus.

Seminal vesicles

The seminal vesicles or glands are two elongated lobular sacs lying lateral to the ampulla of the ductus deferens between the base of the bladder and the rectum (see Fig. 6.13). The seminal gland secretes an alkaline fluid. It joins the lateral side of the ductus deferens, forming the ejaculatory duct.

Ejaculatory ducts

The ejaculatory ducts are formed by the union of the seminal gland and the ductus deferens. They are short, thin-walled tubes that lie almost completely within the prostate and open onto the seminal colliculus within the prostatic utricle.

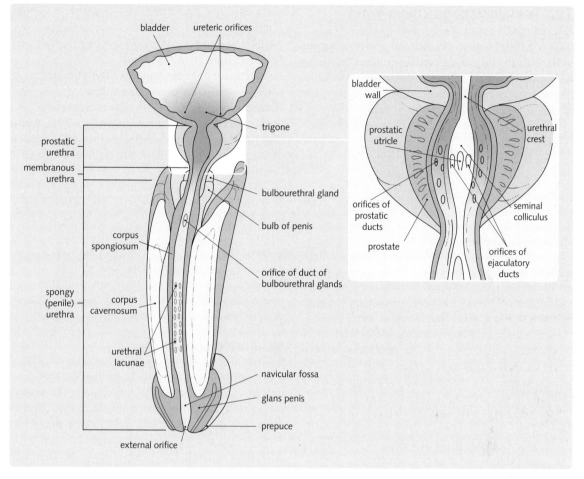

Fig. 6.14 Male urethra (showing details of the prostatic urethra).

Prostate

The prostate is a chestnut-shaped accessory reproductive gland that lies just below the bladder, surrounding the prostatic urethra (see Fig. 6.14). It has a base that is closely related to the bladder, and an apex that is in contact with the sphincter urethrae muscle.

The prostate has right and left lobes united by a fibromuscular isthmus that passes anterior to the urethra. The posterior lobe lies above and behind the lateral lobes.

The prostate is pierced by the proximal urethra.

The fibrous capsule of the prostate completely surrounds the gland, and a thick sheath of visceral pelvic fascia surrounds the capsule and is continuous with the puboprostatic ligaments.

The two are separated by the prostatic plexus of veins.

Blood supply is from the internal pudendal, middle rectal, and inferior vesical arteries. Veins drain to the prostatic plexus, which eventually drains into the internal iliac veins.

Benign prostatic hypertrophy affects almost all elderly males. It may cause urinary obstruction and nocturia. Severe enlargement as well as a prostatic carcinoma require a prostatectomy, which can affect sexual function.

Semen includes secretions of the seminal glands (e.g., vitamin C, fructose) and the prostate (e.g., acid phosphatase) in addition to spermatozoa. This is delivered to the prostatic part of the urethra. A single ejaculate is about 3.0 mL.

The female reproductive tract

Uterus

This is a thick-walled, pear-shaped muscular organ within which the embryo and fetus develop. Most of the wall is smooth muscle, the myometrium. The mucosa is the endometrium.

The uterus has four parts (Fig. 6.15):
- The fundus lies above the entrances of the uterine tubes.
- The body receives the uterine tubes. It is enclosed within a fold of peritoneum, which laterally becomes the double-layered broad ligament. The cavity of the uterus is a mere slit that occupies the body.
- The isthmus is a constricted, short, inferior segment of the uterus which terminates at the internal os.
- The cylindrical cervix is the narrowest part of the uterus. It has a supravaginal part between the isthmus and the vagina and a vaginal part, which protrudes into the vagina. The part of the vagina that surrounds the protruding cervix creates a recess (fornix), which is the deepest posteriorly. The cervical canal is continuous with the uterine cavity at the internal os. It opens into the vagina at the external os.

The cervical canal is lined by columnar epithelium; the vagina is lined by stratified squamous epithelium. Between the two regions is a transition zone where cervical carcinomas can arise. A cervical (Pap) smear attempts to identify premalignant conditions so the suspect area can be removed before cancers arise.

The upper anterior, superior, and posterior surfaces of the uterus are covered by peritoneum. Posteriorly the peritoneum reflects onto the rectum to form the rectouterine pouch (Fig. 6.16). The peritoneum continues from the lateral surface of the uterus to the pelvic side wall as the broad ligament.

The uterus is described as being anteflexed or bent anteriorly on the cervix, and the axis of the cervix is also bent forward on the vagina, or anteverted. Thus the external os faces the posterior wall of the vagina and the posterior fornix is deeper than the lateral or anterior fornices. The uterus leans anteriorly over the empty bladder, but as the bladder fills, the angles of anteflexion and anteversion lessen.

Uterine (fallopian) tubes

The uterine tubes extend laterally from the uterine horns at the junction of the body and fundus of the uterus. They run in the free edge of the broad ligament (see Fig. 6.15). The region of the broad ligament investing each tube is the mesosalpinx.

The uterine tube is composed of:
- The intrauterine part, which passes through the uterine wall.

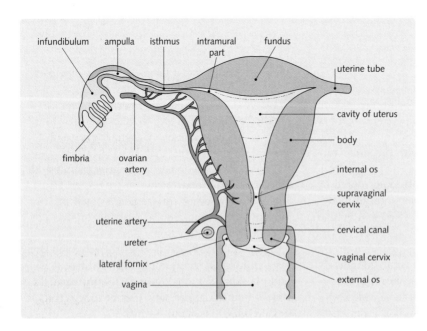

Fig. 6.15 Uterus and its blood supply.

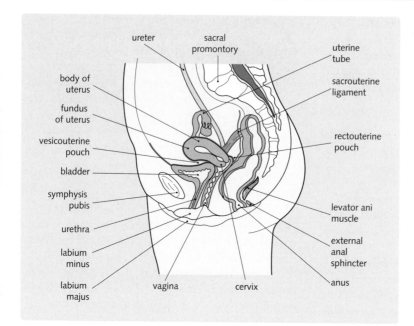

Fig. 6.16 Sagittal section through the female pelvis.

- The isthmus, which enters the uterine horn.
- The ampulla, which is the widest and longest part of the tube.
- The infundibulum, the distal part of the tube with finger-like processes or fimbriae. One of these fimbria, the ovarian fimbria, is attached to the ovary.

When the ovum is shed into the peritoneal cavity, it is trapped by the fimbriae and swept into the ampulla, where fertilization usually occurs. Occasionally the fertilized ovum may implant in the tube or in the peritoneal cavity (an ectopic pregnancy).

Ligaments of the uterus

The broad ligament is a double fold of peritoneum that extends from the lateral uterus to the pelvic side wall (Fig. 6.17). The mesosalpinx is the region within which lie the uterine tubes, the mesometrium encloses the uterus, and the mesovarium is an extension of the posterior layer that encloses the ovary.

The suspensory ligament of the ovary is a fold of peritoneum over the ovarian vessels and lymphatics.

The ligament of the ovary attaches the ovary to the wall of the uterus just below the uterine tube. The round ligament extends from the body of the

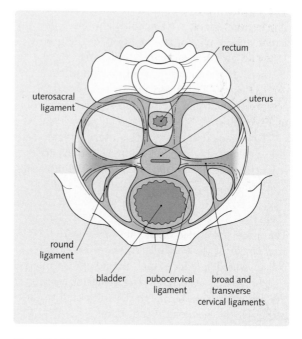

Fig. 6.17 Ligaments of the uterus.

uterus to where the ligament of the ovary attaches to the deep inguinal ring. It passes through the inguinal canal to the labium majus. Both of these ligaments represent remnants of the gubernaculum (see section on the testis).

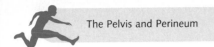

Transverse cervical ligaments (cardinal ligaments) are thickened connective tissue at the base of each broad ligament, extending from the cervix and vaginal fornix to the side wall of the pelvis. They stabilize the cervix laterally.

The uterosacral ligaments extend posterolaterally in the pelvic fascia from the sides of the cervix, passing on either side of the rectum to the middle of the sacrum. They keep the cervix in an upright position.

The pubocervical ligaments are a part of the tendinous arch of the pelvic fascia and extend from the cervix and upper vagina to the posterior aspect of the pubic bones.

The parametrium is the tissue lying between the two peritoneal layers of the broad ligament. It contains the uterine and ovarian vessels and lymphatics, the ligament of the ovary, the round ligament, and the suspensory ligament of the ovary.

Vessels of the uterus and uterine tubes

The uterine artery, a branch of the internal iliac artery, runs along the lateral aspect of the uterus and gives off a vaginal branch within the broad ligament. It anastomoses with branches of the ovarian artery. Each artery gives rise to tubal branches, which anastomose and supply the uterine tubes.

The venous drainage is into a uterine plexus on either side of the cervix. Two uterine veins arise from the plexus, and these drain into the internal iliac vein.

Ovary

The ovary is an ovoid organ that lies near the attachment of the broad ligament to the lateral pelvic walls. It produces the ova and sex hormones.

The ovary is attached to the posterior layer of the broad ligament by the mesovarium and to the uterus by the ligament of the ovary.

Blood supply is from the ovarian artery, a branch of the abdominal aorta. It runs in the suspensory ligament of the ovary, providing branches to the uterus and uterine tubes. It anastomoses with the uterine artery. The veins of an ovarian venous plexus merge to form one vein that follows the artery superiorly. The right ovarian vein drains into the inferior vena cava; the left vein drains into the left renal vein.

The uterine tubes are the most common site of an ectopic pregnancy. If not diagnosed early, tubal rupture and severe hemorrhaging can threaten the mother's life.

Vagina

The vagina is continuous with the cervix at the external os, and it opens into the perineum at the vaginal orifice (see Fig. 6.16). The vaginal fornices surround the part of the cervix that projects into the vagina. The posterior part of the vaginal fornix is deepest and directly related posteriorly to the rectouterine pouch of Douglas. Anteriorly, the vagina is related to the urethra and the bladder, from which it is separated by loose connective tissue.

The superior part of the vagina is supplied by the uterine artery, and the middle and lower parts by vaginal branches of the internal iliac and internal pudendal. The vaginal venous plexus is continuous with the uterine plexus and drains to the internal iliac vein via the uterine vein.

A bimanual vaginal (pelvic exam) can be done through the relatively thin wall of the vagina, with the other hand placing pressure on the lower abdominal wall so that the ovaries can be fully palpated.

Vessels of the pelvis

The pelvic walls and cavity are supplied by branches of the internal iliac arteries, and venous drainage is into the internal iliac veins.

Internal iliac artery

The common iliac artery bifurcates at the pelvic brim opposite the sacroiliac joint into the internal and external iliac arteries (Fig. 6.18). The internal

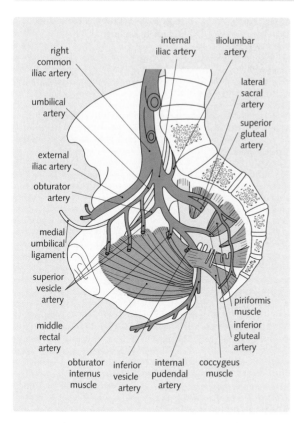

Fig. 6.18 Branches of the internal iliac artery.

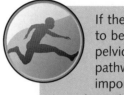

If the internal iliac artery has to be ligated to control a pelvic hemorrhage, collateral pathways become very important, such as the anastomosis between the superior and middle rectal arteries.

Nerves of the pelvis
Obturator nerve

The obturator nerve supplies the adductor compartment of the thigh by emerging from the medial border of psoas and passing along the side of the pelvis to the canal where it supplies the obturator externus and the hip joint. It passes through the obturator foramen into the thigh with the obturator artery and vein below it.

The obturator nerve may be damaged during pelvic surgery, such as ovary removal (oophrectomy). This results in the painful spasms of adductor muscles of the thigh and cutaneous sensory loss over the medial thigh and knee.

iliac artery passes inferiorly and branches into anterior and posterior divisions. The external iliac artery is concerned mainly with the blood supply to the lower limb.

Internal iliac vein

The internal iliac vein commences at the greater sciatic notch and passes superiorly out of the pelvis, posterior to the artery. Here, it joins the external iliac vein at the level of the L4 or L5 veterbra to form the common iliac vein.

Tributaries include:
- Veins corresponding to the arteries.
- The uterine and vesicoprostatic venous plexuses.
- The rectal venous plexuses.
- The lateral sacral veins (it communicates with the vertebral venous plexus via these veins).

There is no umbilical vein.

Sacral plexus

The sacral plexus is formed by the anterior rami of L4 and L5 spinal nerves via the lumbrosacral trunk and the anterior rami of S1–S4 spinal nerves (Fig. 6.19). The plexus lies on the piriformis muscle, and it is covered by the pelvic fascia. The lateral sacral arteries and veins lie over the plexus. The sacral nerves and the lumbosacral trunk combine and then divide into the anterior and posterior divisions.

Sacral sympathetic trunk

The sacral sympathetic trunks are a continuation of the lumbar sympathetic trunks across the pelvic brim. They descend behind the common iliac vessels and then on the pelvic surface of the sacrum, medial to the pelvic sacral foramina. There

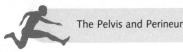

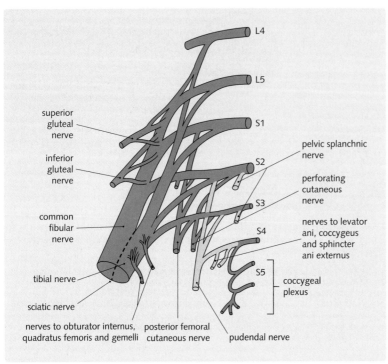

Fig. 6.19 Sacral plexus and its major branches.

are four ganglia along the trunk. The trunks of the two sides unite anterior to the coccyx at a small swelling—the ganglion impar. The sacral sympathetic trunk gives communicating branches via gray rami communicants to the ventral rami of all the sacral nerves and visceral branches (sacral splanchnic nerves) to the inferior hypogastric plexus.

Inferior hypogastric plexus

The right and left hypogastric plexuses comprise the pelvic plexus (Fig. 6.20). Branches of this plexus spread out to form plexuses around the bladder, seminal vesicles and prostate in the male, and the cervix, vagina, and bladder in the female.

The pelvic splanchnic nerves are the sacral parasympathetic outflow from the S2, S3, and S4 spinal cord levels. They run directly from the ventral rami of these nerves to contribute to the pelvic plexus. Together, the autonomic nerves of the pelvis control micturition, defecation, erection, ejaculation, and orgasm. Visceral afferent fibers carrying pain information from the uterus ascend along the right and left hypogastric nerves. Afferent fibers also reach the spinal cord via the pelvic splanchnics.

Lymphatic drainage of the pelvis

This is summarized in Fig. 6.21.

The perineum

The perineum is the narrow region between the proximal thighs, which becomes a diamond shaped area when the thighs are abducted. It is bounded superiorly by the pelvic outlet. Fig. 6.22 illustrates the boundaries of the perineum.

A line drawn between the ischial tuberosities divides the perineum into an anterior urogenital triangle and a posterior anal triangle.

Anal triangle

The anterior boundary of the anal triangle is a transverse line between the ischial tuberosities. The lateral boundaries are the sacrotuberous ligaments and the apex is the tip of the coccyx (see Fig. 6.22). It contains the two ischiorectal fossae separated by, from posterior to anterior, the anococcygeal ligament, the anal canal, and the perineal body. The triangle slopes anteriorly and

124

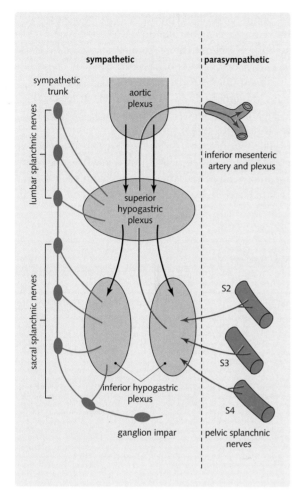

Fig. 6.20 Autonomic plexuses in the pelvis.

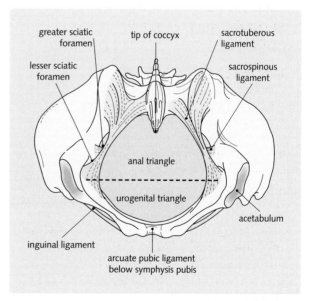

Lymphatic drainage of the pelvis	
Structure	**Lymphatic drainage**
Anal canal	*Above pectinate line:* common iliac and lumbar nodes *Below pectinate line:* superficial inguinal nodes
Bladder	Internal and external iliac nodes
Ovary	Lumbar nodes
Rectum	Inferior mesenteric nodes Internal iliac nodes Pararectal nodes Lumbar nodes
Urethra	Internal iliac nodes Superior inguinal nodes
Uterus and uterine ducts	External iliac nodes Internal iliac nodes Sacral nodes Lumbar nodes
Vagina	Common, internal, and external iliac nodes Superficial inguinal nodes

Fig. 6.21 Lymphatic drainage of the pelvis.

inferiorly from its apex. Muscles of the anal triangle are outlined in Fig. 6.23.

Anal canal
The anal canal commences at the anorectal junction where the rectum is encircled by the puborectalis muscle and descends between the anococcygeal ligament posteriorly and the perineal body anteriorly. It extends for about 3 cm and ends at the anus.

Lining of the anal canal
The upper part of the anal canal is lined by columnar epithelium with goblet cells that is thrown into longitudinal folds—the anal columns. Inferiorly, these columns are linked by horizontal folds, forming the anal valves. The recesses behind the valves are the anal sinuses, where the anal

Fig. 6.22 Boundaries of the perineum, viewed from above.

glands open. The lower margins of the anal valves form the pectinate line. The pectinate line marks the approximate junction of tissue derived from embryonic endoderm and embryonic ectoderm. Thus the anal canal superior to the line differs from that below the line in arterial supply, venous and lymphatic drainage, and innervation (see Fig. 6.25).

Muscular wall of the anal canal

This is composed of internal and external anal sphincters (Fig. 6.24).

The internal anal sphincter is an involuntary muscle that is a continuation of the circular smooth muscle of the rectum. It surrounds the upper three-quarters of the anal canal.

This sphincter is tonically contracted via parasympathetic innervation to prevent leakage: sympathetic innervation relaxes it in response to fecal pressure or gas.

The external anal sphincter has subcutaneous, superficial, and deep parts but these fuse together, forming a single muscular mass. The muscle is striated and under voluntary control. The external

Muscles of the anal triangle			
Name of muscle (nerve supply)	Origin	Insertion	Action
External anal sphincter: subcutaneous part (inferior rectal nerve and perineal branch of fourth sacral nerve)	Encircles anal canal, no bony attachments		Voluntary sphincter of anal canal
External anal sphincter: superficial part (inferior rectal nerve and perineal branch of fourth sacral nerve)	Perineal body	Coccyx	Voluntary sphincter of anal canal
External anal sphincter: deep part (inferior rectal nerve and perineal branch of fourth sacral nerve)	Encircles anal canal	Coccyx	Voluntary sphincter of anal canal

Fig. 6.23 Muscles of the anal triangle.

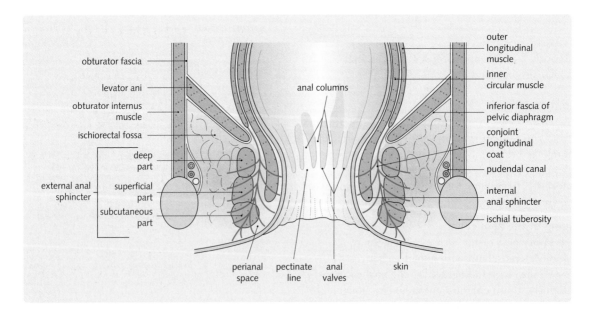

Fig. 6.24 Anal canal and ischiorectal fossa.

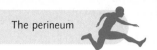

sphincter is supplied by the perineal branch of S4 spinal nerve and the inferior rectal nerve (from the pudendal nerve). Voluntary contraction of the sphincter delays defecation.

Fig. 6.25 shows the blood supply and lymphatic drainage of the anal canal.

Ischioanal (ischiorectal) fossa and pudendal canal

The ischiorectal fossae are wedge-shaped spaces between the skin of the anal region and the pelvic diaphragm, which encircle the anal canal. They are filled with adipose tissue, traversed by fibrous bands, which enables the fat to support the anal canal but be displaced by expansion of the canal during defecation. On the lateral walls of the fossae are found the pudendal canals within which are the internal pudendal vessels and pudendal nerves. These give rise to the inferior rectal arteries and nerves before entering the canal (see Fig. 6.24). The boundaries of the ischiorectal fossa are detailed in Fig. 6.26.

The pudendal canal lies on the lateral wall of the ischiorectal fossa—the inner surface of the ischial tuberosity. The canal is enclosed by fascia that is continuous with the obturator internus fascia above, and that fuses with the ischial tuberosity below. It contains the internal pudendal vessels and the pudendal nerve, which exit the pelvic cavity via the greater sciatic forament, wrap around the ischial spine and pass through the lesser sciatic foramen to enter the pudendal canal, and from there pass to the superficial perineal pouch (space).

Blood supply and lymphatic drainage of the anal canal

Arterial supply	Origin
Above pectinate line: Superior rectal artery	Inferior mesenteric artery
Below pectinate line: Inferior rectal artery	Internal pudendal artery
Connecting: Middle rectal artery	Internal iliac artery
Venous drainage	**Destination**
Above pectinate line: Internal venous plexus	Superior rectal veins
Muscular coat of upper canal	Middle rectal veins
Below pectinate line: External venous plexus	Inferior rectal veins
Lymphatic drainage	**Destination**
Above pectinate line	Internal iliac nodes
Below pectinate line	Superficial inguinal nodes
Innervation	**Destination**
Above pectinate line	Pelvis plexus (sympathetic and parasympathetic)
Below pectinate line	Inferior rectal nerve (somatic from pudendal nerve)

Fig. 6.25 Blood supply and lymphatic drainage of the anal canal.

 The fat of the ischiorectal fossa has a poor blood supply. Therefore, it is vulnerable to infection and abscess formation.

Boundaries of the ischiorectal fossa

Boundary	Components
Base	Skin over anal region of perineum
Medial wall	Anal canal and external anal sphincter; levator ani descends to sphincter
Lateral wall	Ischial tuberosity and obturator internus; covered by obturator fascia
Apex	Where levator ani is attached to the tendinous origins over obturator fascia
Anterior extension	Superior to deep perineal pouch
Posterior extension	Sacrotuberous ligaments and gluteus maximus

Fig. 6.26 Boundaries of the ischiorectal fossa.

The male urogenital triangle

The male urogenital triangle is bounded posteriorly by a transverse line between the two ischial tuberosities. Its lateral boundaries are the ischiopubic rami, which meet at the apex—the pubic symphysis (see Fig. 6.22).

Within the urogenital triangle is the deep perineal space. The space lies below the anterior extent of the levator ani muscle. The deep perineal space is open superiorly, bounded only by loose pelvic fascia. Inferiorly it is bounded by a tough, fibrous membrane, the perineal membrane, which is attached to the ischiopubic rami from just posterior to the pubic symphysis to the ischial tuberosities (Fig. 6.27).

The deep space contains the deep transverse perineal muscles and the sphincter urethrae.

A superficial perineal fascia layer that is continuous with the membranous superficial fascia (Scarpa's fascia) of the anterior abdominal wall descends and lines the scrotum, where it is called the dartos layer, because it contains the dartos muscle that is attached to the skin. Between this superficial perineal fascia (Colles') and perineal membrane is the superficial perineal space.

The urethra traverses the deep perineal space and perineal membrane (see Fig. 6.27).

Fig. 6.28 outlines the muscles of the urogenital triangle. These muscles are involved in micturition, copulation, and support of the pelvic viscera.

Deep perineal space

The deep perineal space is the region above the perineal membrane. It contains the deep transverse perineal muscles and sphincter urethrae and the following structures:
- The membranous urethra.
- The bulbourethral glands (male).
- Related vessels from the internal pudendal artery and vein.
- The dorsal nerve of the penis.

The bulbourethral glands are two small glands lying on either side of the membranous urethra (see Fig. 6.26). Their ducts pierce the perineal membrane to enter the spongy part of the urethra. Secretions contribute to the seminal fluid.

Superficial perineal space

The superficial perineal space is bounded inferiorly by the superficial perineal fascia, a continuation of the membranous superficial fascia of the anterior abdominal wall. It is attached to the ischiopubic rami, the posterior border of the perineal membrane, the perineal body, and the fascia lata of

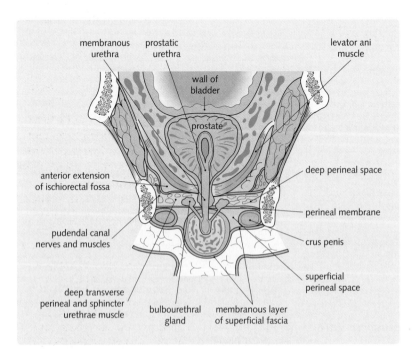

Fig. 6.27 Coronal section of the male perineum.

Muscles of the urogenital triangle			
Name of muscle (nerve supply)	Origin	Insertion	Action
Superficial transverse perineal muscle (deep perineal branch of pudendal nerve)	Ischial tuberosity	Perineal body	Fixes perineal body to support pelvic viscera and resist intra-abdominal pressure
Bulbospongiosus (deep perineal branch of pudendal nerve)	Perineal body and median raphe in male, perineal body in female	Fascia of bulb of penis and corpora spongiosum and cavernosum in male; fascia of bulbs of vestibule in female	In male, empties urethra after micturition and ejaculation and assists in erection of penis; in female, sphincter of vagina and assists in erection of clitoris
Ischiocavernosus (deep perineal branch of pudendal nerve)	Ischial tuberosities and ischio-pubic rami in male and female	Crura of penis or clitoris	Erection of penis or clitoris
Deep transverse perineal muscle (deep perineal branch of pudendal nerve)	Ischiopubic rami and ischial tuberosities	Perineal body	Fixes perineal body to support pelvic viscera and resist intra-abdominal pressure
Sphincter urethrae (deep perineal branch of pudendal nerve)	Ishiopubic ramus and ischial tuberosities	Surrounds urethra, ascends to prostate in males and vagina in females	Compresses urethra to maintain continence

Fig. 6.28 Muscles of the urogenital triangle.

the thigh. The superficial perineal fascia (Colles') extends into the penis as the superficial fascia of the penis and into the scrotum as the dartos tunic.

Superiorly the space is limited by the perineal membrane. The contents of the space include the proximal spongy urethra, the root of the penis (bulb and crura), and superficial transverse perineal, bulbospongiosus, and ischiocavernosus muscles. It also contains the perineal branches of the internal pudendal artery and pudendal nerve.

Rupture of the penile urethra causes urine to leak into the superficial perineal space. Due to the superficial perineal fascia's continuity with the anterior abdominal wall and penile and scrotal superficial fascia, urine can swell the scrotum and penis and pass upward into the anterior abdominal wall.

The male external genitalia

The male external genitalia consist of the penis and the scrotum. The scrotum is described in Chapter 5.

Penis

The penis is the male copulatory organ. It consists of the root, the body, and the glans (Fig. 6.29).

The root is made up of three masses of erectile tissue: the bulb of the penis and the right and left crura. The posterior part of the bulb is penetrated by the urethra. The bulb and crura are surrounded by the bulbospongiosus and ischiocavernosus muscles, respectively. Each crus is directly related to the inner surface of an inferior ischial ramus.

The crura become the corpora cavernosa; the bulb becomes the corpus spongiosum. The urethra passes into the erectile tissue of the bulb, and it continues in the corpus spongiosum to the external urethral orifice.

The distal end of the corpus spongiosum expands to form the glans penis. The glans has a marginal projection at its proximal end called the

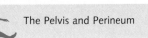

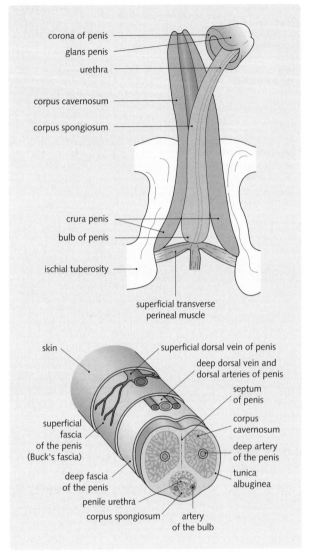

corona of penis
glans penis
urethra

corpus cavernosum

corpus spongiosum

crura penis

bulb of penis

ischial tuberosity

superficial transverse
perineal muscle

skin

superficial dorsal vein of penis

deep dorsal vein and
dorsal arteries of penis

septum
of penis

corpus
cavernosum

superficial
fascia
of the penis
(Buck's fascia)

deep artery
of the penis

tunica
albuginea

deep fascia
of the penis

penile urethra

corpus spongiosum   artery
of the bulb

Fig. 6.29 Composition and structure of the penis.

the tunica albuginea. External to this deep fascia is the superficial fascia of the penis.

The corpus spongiosum, spongy urethra, and corpora cavernosa receive blood from the deep arteries of the penis. The bulb and urethra are supplied by the artery to the bulb and the dorsal artery. The dorsal artery supplies the skin and superficial fascial layers as well.

The deep arteries of the penis give off numerous branches to the cavernous spaces that allow rapid distension of the cavernous spaces to produce an erection. These branches, called helicine arteries, are highly coiled when the penis is flaccid.

Venous drainage is from the cavernous spaces via a venous plexus to the deep dorsal vein, which drains to the prostatic venous plexus.

Parasympathetic fibers enter the penis from the prostatic nerve plexus and innervate the smooth muscle of the helicine arteries, causing them to relax and straighten and allowing blood to flow into the cavernous spaces, with a resulting erection. Sensory and sympathetic innervation is provided by the pudendal nerve via its terminal branch, the dorsal nerve of the penis. Ejaculation is a sympathetic response.

 To recall the role of autonomic innervation in the male sexual response, remember point (parasympathetic) and shoot (sympathetic).

corona of the glans. The body is surrounded by thin loose skin and contains no muscle. At the proximal part of the glans penis the skin is reflected upon itself to form a double layer called the prepuce or foreskin, which covers the glans. The prepuce is attached to the ventral surface of the glans by a fold of skin, the frenulum of the prepuce, which contains a small artery.

A tough tunica albuginea surrounds and passes trabeculae into the three corpora, forming numerous spaces into which arteries empty. The deep fascia of the penis (Buck's fascia) encircles

Vessels of the male urogenital triangle
The internal pudendal artery is a branch of the internal iliac artery. Its course, distribution, and branches are outlined in Fig. 6.30.

The internal pudendal veins accompany the arteries. The deep dorsal vein of the penis drains into the prostatic plexus. The superficial dorsal vein of the penis drains to an external pudendal vein and then to the femoral vein.

The blood supply to the scrotum is described in Chapter 5.

Lymphatics of the male urogenital triangle
Lymph from the skin of the penis and scrotum drains into the superficial inguinal nodes.

Internal pudendal artery and its branches		
Vessel	**Source**	**Course and distribution**
Internal pudendal artery	Anterior division of internal iliac artery	Exits the pelvis via the greater sciatic foramen, hooks around the ischial spine, and enters the perineum via the lesser sciatic foramen and the pudendal canal. At the anterior end the canal branches enter the superficial and deep perineal pouches
Inferior rectal artery	Internal pudendal artery	Arises at the entrance of the inguinal canal, crosses the ischiorectal fossa to supply the external anal sphincter and skin of the anal canal below the pectineal line
Perineal branch	Internal pudendal artery	Passes to the superficial perineal space to supply its superficial perineal muscles and the scrotum (or vestibule in female)
Artery to bulb of penis (or clitoris)	Internal pudendal artery	Pierces the perineal membrane to supply the erectile tissue of the bulb of the penis and the bulbourethral glands (male) or bulb of the vestibule and the bulbourethral glands (female)
Deep artery of penis (or clitoris)	Internal pudendal artery	Passes through the perineal membrane to supply the corpus cavernosum
Dorsal artery of penis (or clitoris)	Internal pudendal artery	Passes through the deep pouch to the dorsum of the penis (or clitoris). It supplies the erectile tissue of the corpus cavernosum and glans
Urethral artery	Internal pudendal artery	Supplies the urethra

Fig. 6.30 Internal pudendal artery and its branches.

Lymphatics from the substance of the penis are tributaries of the deep inguinal and external and internal iliac nodes.

Nerves of the male urogenital triangle

The pudendal nerve (S2–S4) passes with the internal pudendal artery through the lesser sciatic foramen and, just before entering the pudendal canal, it gives rise to the inferior rectal nerve. The inferior rectal nerve supplies the external anal sphincter and the skin around the anus. Approaching the posterior border of the perineal membrane, the nerve divides into the perineal nerve and the dorsal nerve of the penis. The perineal nerve breaks up into muscular branches to the remaining striated muscles of the perineum and sensory branches, and posterior scrotal or posterior labial nerves.

The dorsal nerve of the penis runs with the dorsal artery of the penis. It passes over the dorsum of the penis lateral to the artery and terminates in the glans.

The suspensory ligament of the penis is composed of deep fascia from the pubic symphysis that descends and splits to encircle the penis at the junction of its body and root. The fundiform ligament of the penis is composed of loose collagen and elastic fibers from the linea alba that descend and divide, passing on either side of the penis and blending with the dartos fascia of the scrotum.

The nerve supply to the scrotum is described in Chapter 5.

To recall the pudendal nerve supplies levator ani, remember S2, 3, 4 keeps the perineum off the floor.

The female urogenital triangle

The muscles, fasciae, and spaces of the female urogenital triangle are similar to those of the male urogenital triangle. However, certain features differ because of the presence of the vagina and external female genitalia.

The deep perineal space differs from that of the male in that the vagina traverses it, and it lacks the female equivalent of the bulbourethral gland.

The superficial perineal space again is similar to that of the male, and it is lined by a less-defined superficial perineal fascia. However, it differs in that it contains the following:

- Vagina.
- Bulbs of the vestibule and their surrounding muscle.
- Greater vestibular glands.
- A considerable amount of fat.

Perineal membrane
The perineal membrane is wider in the female since the pelvis is wider, and it is also somewhat weakened because the vagina pierces it. As the urethra and vagina traverse the membrane their outer fascial covering fuses with it.

Perineal body
In the female, the perineal body lies between the vagina and the anal canal. The perineal body is larger in females and has greater mobility. The superficial and deep transverse perineal muscles, the pubovaginalis, bulbospongiosus, and the superficial part of the external anal sphincter are attached to the perineal body.

The external female genitalia
The external female genitalia consist of the mons pubis, clitoris, vagina, vestibule, external urethral orifice, labia majora, and labia minora. Together these parts form the vulva (Fig. 6.31).

Mons pubis
In the adult (i.e., after puberty), this is a mound of coarse-haired skin with subcutaneous fat anterior to the pubic symphysis. The mons pubis extends posteriorly as the labia majora.

Labia majora
These two fatty folds of skin are filled with subcutaneous fat and are the homologs of the two halves of the scrotal sac. They meet anteriorly to form the anterior commissure, and they are continuous with the mons pubis. As the folds pass posteriorly they fade into the skin near the anus. This area is the posterior commissure. The round ligament of the uterus ends in the labium majus.

Labia minora
These are fat-free skin folds that lie within the labia majora and surround the vestibule of the vagina. They enclose the clitoris by dividing into upper and lower folds. The upper folds from either side fuse to form the prepuce anteriorly and lower folds fuse to form the frenulum posteriorly.

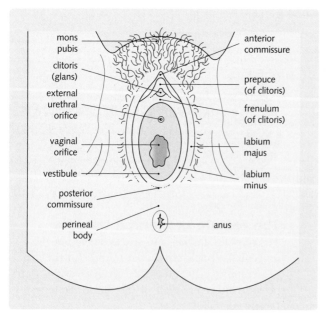

Fig. 6.31 Female external genitalia.

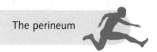

Clitoris
This homolog of the penis consists of two crura attached to the perineal membrane and ischiopubic rami. Anteriorly, the crura become the corpora cavernosa. These are bound together by fascia to form the body of the clitoris. The body ends at a tiny glans.

Vestibule
This contains the openings of the greater vestibular glands and the vagina, and the external urethral orifice.

Bulbs of the vestibule
These are homologs of the penile bulb and the proximal corpora cavernosa. Posteriorly these two erectile masses, located on either side of the vagina and urethra, are attached to the perineal membrane. Anteriorly they taper to join the glans of the clitoris. Each is covered by the bulbospongiosus muscle.

Greater vestibular glands
The homologs of the bulbourethral glands, they are found in the superficial perineal pouch in contact with the posterior end of the bulb of the vestibule. Their ducts open into the vestibule and lubricate the vagina in sexual arousal.

Vagina
The vagina passes inferiorly through the pelvic floor surrounded by the pubococcygeous and the puborectalis; anteriorly, it is closely related to the urethra; posteriorly, the perineal body separates it from the anal canal; inferiorly, it opens into the vestibule. This opening is partially occluded by a thin mucous membrane—the hymen—which is usually destroyed during sexual intercourse.

External urethral orifice
This lies in the vestibule posterior to the glans of the clitoris but anterior to the vaginal opening.

Lymphatics of the female urogenital triangle
The lymph drains to the superficial inguinal lymph nodes.

Vessels and nerves of the female urogenital triangle
The internal pudendal artery has a similar course and distribution in the female as in the male, except:
- Posterior labial branches replace scrotal branches.
- The artery to the bulb and vestibule and the dorsal arteries of the clitoris replace the arteries to the penile bulb and penis.

The blood supply to the external genitalia (e.g., the labia and vestibule) is the same as the scrotum. Superficial and deep external pudendal arteries from the femoral artery supply them. Corresponding veins drain to the great saphenous vein. The pudendal nerve has a similar distribution in both genders. The only difference is in the naming of the nerves, in which labial replaces scrotal.

The nerve supply to the labia is the same as for the scrotum:
- The anterior third is supplied by the ilioinguinal nerve and the genital branch of the genitofemoral nerve.
- The posterior two-thirds are supplied by the posterior deep and superficial labial branches of the pudendal nerve (medially) and by the perineal branch of the posterior femoral cutaneous nerve (laterally).

The pudendal nerve is the principal nerve of the perineum.

A pudendal nerve block relieves pain caused by perineal stretching in childbirth. The anesthetic is injected near the nerve as it crosses the sacrospinous ligament near the ischial spine, which is palpable on vaginal examination. The needle may be passed through the skin or the vaginal wall.

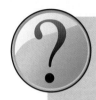

- Describe the surface landmarks of the pelvic bones.
- List the structures palpable on a rectal examination in males and females.
- What are the main features of the pelvic bones and joints, including the position of the pelvis?
- Discuss the differences between male and female pelves.
- Discuss the anatomy of the pelvic floor and wall muscles.
- What is the perineal body and its function?
- Describe the folds and pouches of the peritoneum in the pelvis.
- Describe the anatomy of the rectum.
- What is the course of the ureters in the pelvis?
- Describe the vascular and nerve supply to the ureter.
- Describe the anatomy of the bladder.
- Describe the anatomy of the male reproductive tract.
- Describe the anatomy of the female reproductive tract.
- Outline the vessels of the pelvis.
- Outline the nerves of the pelvis.
- List the lymphatic drainage of the pelvic viscera.
- Describe how the perineum is divided into triangles. What are their contents?
- List the boundaries and contents of the ischioanal fossa.
- Discuss the anatomy of the anal canal, with respect to the pectinate line.
- Describe how the superficial perineal space is formed and its contents in male and female.
- Discuss the path of extravasated urine in the superficial perineal space.
- Describe the male external genitalia.
- Describe the female external genitalia.

7. The Lower Limb

Regions and components of the lower limb

The lower limb is built for support, locomotion, and the maintenance of equilibrium. Weight is transferred from the rigid bony pelvis, through the acetabulum, to the femur. The lower limb has four regions:

- Hip, including the gluteal region.
- Thigh, between the hip and the knee.
- Leg, between the knee and the ankle.
- Foot.

The hip joint is formed by the acetabulum and the head of the femur. It is a very stable joint, with a good range of movement.

The femur articulates with the tibia at the knee joint. Only flexion and extension are possible at this joint. The superior part of the fibula serves for muscle attachment only, and it does not take part in the formation of the knee joint or in weightbearing. Weight is transferred from the femur to the tibia at the knee joint and from the knee to the ankle joint by the tibia.

Both the tibia and the fibula articulate with the talus to form the ankle joint, where dorsiflexion and plantarflexion movements may occur, with a small amount of rotation, abduction, and adduction.

The blood supply to the lower limb is from the external iliac artery. This becomes the femoral artery beneath the inguinal ligament, and it supplies the entire thigh region. Behind the knee the femoral artery becomes the popliteal artery, which supplies the leg and the foot.

The gluteal region is supplied by the superior and inferior gluteal arteries, branches of the internal iliac artery.

The lower limb is innervated by the lumbar and sacral plexuses via the femoral, obturator, and sciatic nerves. The gluteal region is also supplied by the superior and inferior gluteal nerves.

Surface anatomy and superficial structures

Hip and thigh region

The iliac crest and iliac spines should be familiar (Chapter 6). The greater trochanter of the femur can be palpated on the lateral thigh, about 10 cm below the iliac crest, when the thigh is passively abducted to relax the gluteus medius and minimus.

The large quadriceps muscle makes up the anterior surface of the thigh. It inserts into the patella and, via the patellar ligament, into the tibial tuberosity. The patella is a sesamoid bone into which the quadriceps tendon inserts. It can be easily palpated during flexion and extension.

The iliotibial tract lies on the lateral surface of the thigh. The gluteus maximus and tensor fasciae latae insert into it. It can be demonstrated by raising the leg in an extended position, when it becomes prominent just posterior to the patella on the lateral side.

The hamstrings lie in the posterior compartment of the thigh. They can be demonstrated by attempting to flex the knees against resistance.

Knee region

On the lateral side of the knee the head of the fibula is palpable. The lateral and medial femoral condyles are subcutaneous and the medial in particular can be easily palpated during flexion and extension. The tibial condyles can be palpated on either side of the patellar ligament. Posteriorly, the diamond-shaped popliteal fossa is seen when the knees are flexed against resistance.

Leg region

The subcutaneous anteromedial surface of the tibia (shin bone) is easily felt.

Just below the head of the fibula the common fibular nerve becomes superficial as it runs from the popliteal fossa into the lateral compartment of the leg. It is vulnerable to injury at this point. The fibular muscles comprise the lateral aspect of the leg.

135

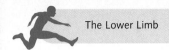

The large gastrocnemius and soleus muscles are seen at the back of the leg. These join to form the tendocalcaneus, which inserts into the posterior calcaneum.

Ankle

The malleoli are prominences medially and laterally. The head of the talus can be palpated anterior to the lateral and medial malleoli when the foot is inverted and everted, respectively.

Superficial veins

The foot drains into the dorsal venous arch, which drains laterally into the small saphenous vein and medially into the great saphenous vein.

Great saphenous vein

The great saphenous vein passes anterior to the medial malleolus, and it ascends in the subcutaneous tissue on the medial side of the leg then posterior to the medial femoral condyle and superior from the adductor tubercle to the saphenous opening in the fascia lata (Fig. 7.1A and inset). Here, it perforates the cribriform fascia covering the opening and joins the femoral vein. It communicates with the deep veins via perforating veins.

The great saphenous vein is valved, allowing flow of blood in one direction only. Damage to the valves may result in varicose veins. The perforating veins also have valves.

Tributaries of the great saphenous vein arise at its proximal end from the anterior and medial aspects of the thigh and from the anterior abdominal wall. These include:

- The superficial circumflex iliac vein.
- The superficial epigastric vein.
- The external pudendal vein.

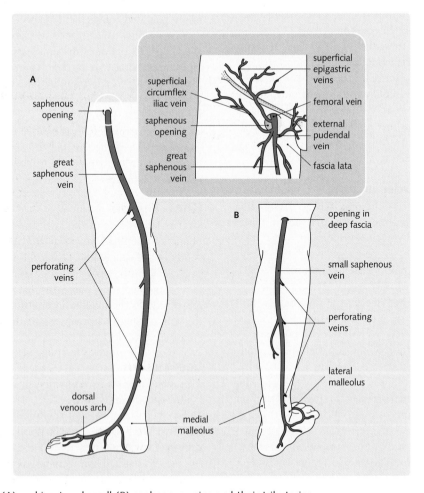

Fig. 7.1 Great (A) and inset and small (B) saphenous veins and their tributaries.

The great saphenous vein is commonly used as a site for cannulation and it may also be used as a graft for a coronary artery bypass operation.

Small (lesser) saphenous vein

The small saphenous vein passes posteriorly to the lateral malleolus and runs superiorly and posteriorly to pierce the deep fascia of the popliteal fossa between the heads of the gastrocnemius, where it joins the popliteal vein (Fig. 7.1B). It drains the lateral part of the leg, and it communicates with the deep veins of the leg via perforating veins.

Lymphatic drainage of the lower limb

Lymphatics from the superficial tissues of the lower limb accompany the great saphenous vein and drain to the superficial inguinal lymph nodes (Fig. 7.2). These nodes lie superficial to the deep fascia around the termination of the saphenous vein. They also receive lymph from the lower part of the perineum, the abdominal wall, and the buttock, and drain to the deep inguinal and external iliac nodes. Lymphatics also accompany the small saphenous vein and drain to nodes

surrounding the popliteal vein in the popliteal fossa.

The deep nodes lie alongside the femoral vein and its tributaries, and they drain the deep tissues of the lower limb. From the leg, lymphatics enter the popliteal nodes and thence to the deep inguinal nodes and finally into nodes lying alongside the external iliac vessels.

Enlarged superficial inguinal nodes indicate disease: to determine the cause, remember that they drain the lower limb and perineum, buttock, and the anterior abdominal wall below the umbilicus. All of these regions must be examined.

Deep and superficial fascia of the lower limb

The membranous superficial fascia (Scarpa's fascia) of the abdomen becomes fused with the deep fascia or fascia lata of the thigh a finger's breadth below the inguinal ligament. Remember, this fusion prevents extravasated fluid (e.g., urine) in the superficial perineal pouch from tracking inferiorly in the lower limb.

The subcutaneous fatty layer of the superficial fascia of the thigh contains the cutaneous nerves, lymphatics, and superficial veins.

The deep fascia of the lower limb, called the fascia lata in the thigh and the crural fascia in the leg, is a dense layer of connective tissue that surrounds the muscles.

The fascia lata prevents bulging of the muscles during contraction and this makes muscular contraction more efficient in pumping blood from the lower limb back to the heart.

Cutaneous innervation of the lower limb

Figs. 7.3 and 7.4 illustrate the dermatomes and cutaneous innervation of the lower limb, respectively.

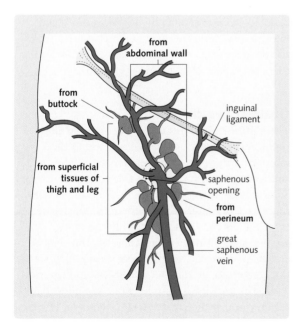

Fig. 7.2 Superficial inguinal lymph nodes.

lower limbs via the hip joint and femur (see Chapter 6).

Femur

The femur is the long bone of the thigh. The bone and its muscle attachments are illustrated in Fig. 7.5.

Fascia lata

The fascia lata is the deep fascia of the thigh. It lies below the skin and superficial fascia, and it encloses the compartments of the thigh. Its attachments can be traced along the pelvis:

- Coccyx, sacrum, sacrotuberous ligament, and ischial tuberosity (posteriorly)
- Pubic tubercle, body of the pubis, and pubic arch (anteriorly)
- Iliac crest (laterally and posteriorly).

Inferiorly the fascia lata is attached to the tibia and fibula and continues below into the deep fascia of the leg (crural fascia).

The iliotibial tract is a thickening of the fascia lata by the addition of longitudinal fibers. It begins at the level of the iliac tubercle and it extends to a tubercle (Gerdy's) on the lateral condyle of the tibia. It encloses the tensor fascia lata muscle and fibers of the gluteus maximus insert into its posterior margin.

The thigh is divided into anterior, posterior, and adductor compartments by lateral, medial, and intermediate intermuscular septa that arise from the deep surface of the fascia lata and attach to the linea aspera of the femur (Fig. 7.6).

Gluteal region

The gluteal region, or buttock, lies behind the pelvis and extends from the iliac crest to the inferior border of the gluteus maximus. The greater and lesser sciatic foramina in this region are formed anteriorly by the greater and lesser sciatic notches, respectively. Posteriorly the foramina are formed from the notches by the sacrotuberous and sacrospinous ligaments. The muscles, the vessels, and the nerves that supply the gluteal region via the greater sciatic foramen are shown in Figs. 7.7–7.10. The piriformis muscle enters the gluteal region through the greater sciatic foramen, filling it, and vessels and nerves either pass superior or inferior to it.

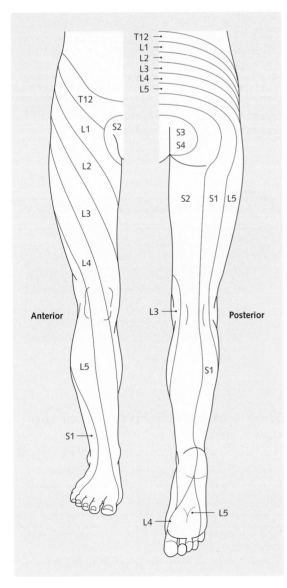

Fig. 7.3 Dermatomes of the lower limb.

The gluteal region, hip, and thigh

Skeleton of the hip and thigh

Pelvic girdle

The pelvic girdle protects the pelvic cavity and supports the body weight. It transmits load to the

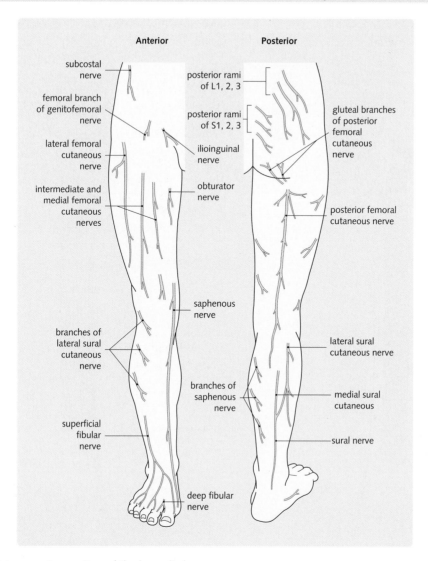

Fig. 7.4 Cutaneous innervation of the lower limb.

The actions of the gluteus medius and minimus are crucial for walking. When one foot is off the ground, the collapse of the pelvis on the side where it is not supported is prevented by contraction of these two muscles on the contralateral side.

The gluteal region is a common site for intramuscular injections. The sciatic nerve is at risk of damage unless injections are given in the upper outer quadrant behind the anterior superior iliac spine and below the iliac crest.

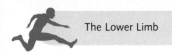

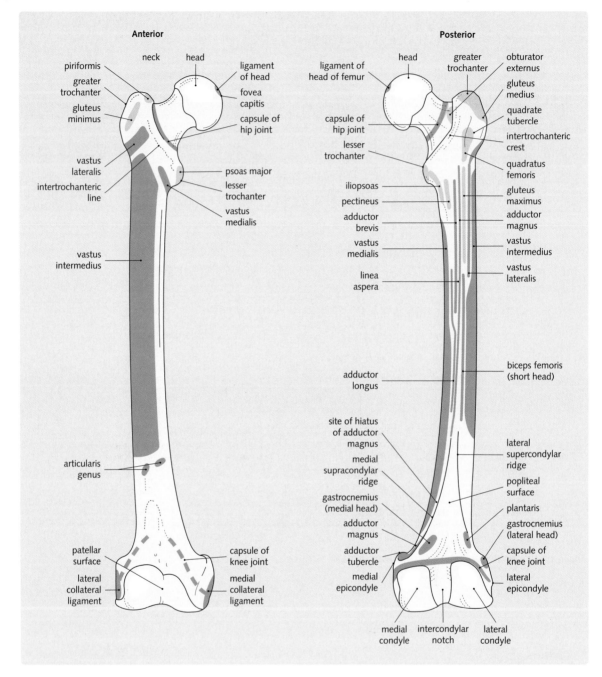

Fig. 7.5 Muscles and ligaments of the anterior and posterior surfaces of the right femur. Light blue = distal attachment; dark blue = proximal attachment.

Fig. 7.6 Compartments of the thigh.

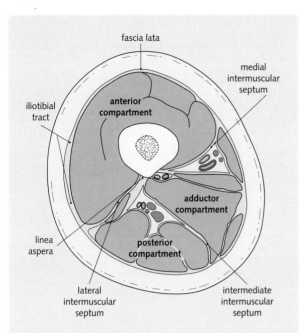

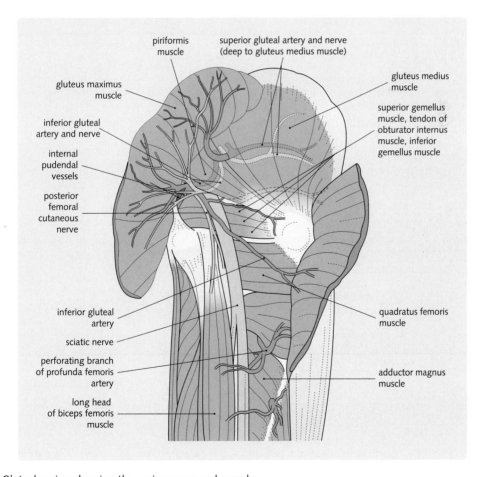

Fig. 7.7 Gluteal region showing the main nerves and vessels.

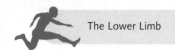

Muscles of the gluteal region

Name of muscle (nerve supply)	Origin	Insertion	Action
Gluteus maximus (inferior gluteal nerve)	External ilium posterior to posterior gluteal line, dorsal sacrum, coccyx, and sacrotuberous ligament	Iliotibial tract and gluteal tuberosity of femur	Extension and lateral rotation of thigh at hip joint
Gluteus medius (superior gluteal nerve)	External ilium between anterior and posterior gluteal lines	Lateral surface of greater trochanter of femur	Abduction and medial rotation of the thigh; keeps pelvis level when walking
Gluteus minimus (superior gluteal nerve)	External ilium between anterior and inferior gluteal lines	Anterior surface of greater trochanter of femur	Abduction and medial rotation of the thigh; keeps pelvis level when walking
Piriformis (S1, S2 nerves)	Anterior surface of sacrum, sacrotuberous ligament	Superior surface of greater trochanter of femur	Rotates thigh laterally at hip joint and stabilizes head of the femur in the acetabulum
Obturator internus (nerve to obturator internus)	Inner surface of obturator membrane and surrounding bone	Medial surface of greater trochanter of femur	Same as above
Gemellus inferior (nerve to the quadratus femoris)	Ischial tuberosity	Medial surface of greater trochanter of femur	Same as above
Gemellus superior (nerve to obturator internus)	Ischial spine	Medial surface of greater trochanter of femur	Same as above
Quadratus femoris (nerve to the quadratus femoris)	Lateral border of the ischial tuberosity	Intertrochanteric crest of femur	Same as above

Fig. 7.8 Muscles of the gluteal region.

Arteries of the gluteal region

Artery	Course and distribution
Internal pudendal	Passes through the greater sciatic foramen inferior to the piriformis to enter the gluteal region, then passes into the perineum via the lesser sciatic foramen; supplies the muscles of the perineum and the external genitalia
Superior gluteal	Enters the gluteal region through the greater sciatic foramen superior to the piriformis; supplies the gluteal maximus, medius, and minimus and tensor fasciae latae
Inferior gluteal	Passes through the greater sciatic foramen inferior to the piriformis to enter the glutal region; supplies gluteus maximus, obturator internus, superior hamstrings, and quadratus femoris

Fig. 7.9 Arteries of the gluteal region.

Nerves of the gluteal region	
Nerve (origin)	**Course and distribution**
Inferior gluteal (anterior rami of L5–S2)	Leaves pelvis through greater sciatic foramen below piriformis and supplies gluteus maximus
Superior gluteal (anterior rami of L4–S1)	Leaves pelvis through greater sciatic foramen above piriformis and passes between gluteus medius and minimus to supply these muscles and tensor fasciae latae
Nerve to quadratus femoris (anterior rami of L4, L5, and S1)	Leaves pelvis through greater sciatic foramen below piriformis to supply hip joint, inferior gemellus, and quadratus femoris
Posterior femoral cutaneous (sacral plexus—S1–S3)	Leaves pelvis through greater sciatic foramen below piriformis, runs deep to gluteus maximus, and emerges from its inferior border to supply skin of lateral perineum, upper medial thigh, and buttock and then surface skin over posterior of calf and thigh
Pudendal (anterior rami of S2–S4)	Enters gluteal region through greater sciatic foramen below piriformis, descends posterior to sacrospinous ligament, enters perineum through lesser sciatic foramen, and supplies the latter
Sciatic (sacral plexus—L4–S3)	Leaves pelvis through greater sciatic foramen below piriformis to enter gluteal region—it has no motor branches in the gluteal region

Fig. 7.10 Nerves of the gluteal region.

Anterior compartment of the thigh

The anterior compartment of the thigh is bound anterolaterally by the fascia lata. The medial intermuscular septum separates it from the medial compartment, and the lateral intermuscular septum, the strongest of the septa, separates the anterior compartment from the posterior compartment.

The muscles of the anterior compartment are described in Fig. 7.11.

Factors stabilizing the patella

The pull of the quadriceps tendon is slightly oblique, while the pull of the patella ligament is vertical. Thus the patella has the tendency to move laterally. This is prevented by:

- The lateral condyle of the femur has a longer anterior prominence (see Fig. 7.20)
- The lowest fibers of vastus medialis insert into the patella directly, and they are approximately horizontal. Contraction pulls the patella medially.

The patella also provides additional leverage for the quadriceps by moving the tendon further from the joint axis.

Femoral triangle

The femoral triangle is a triangular fascial space bounded by the:

- Inguinal ligament superiorly.
- Adductor longus muscle medially.
- Sartorius muscle laterally.

It contains the femoral artery, vein, and nerve and their branches or tributaries (Fig. 7.12). These all lie superficially just beneath the skin, superficial fascia, and fascia lata.

The femoral artery and vein and the femoral canal are enclosed by the femoral sheath, which is a continuation of the transversalis and iliopsoas fasciae into the thigh. The fascia of the isopsoas muscle is thickened on its anteromedial surface, where it is called the iliopectineal arch. This separates the space under the inguinal ligament into a medial vascular compartment containing the femoral sheath and its contents, and the femoral branch of the genitofemoral nerve, and a lateral muscular compartment, containing the ilopsoas muscle and the femoral nerve in the fascia on its surface.

143

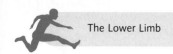
Muscles of the anterior compartment of the thigh

Name of muscle	Origin	Insertion	Action
Tensor fasciae latae (superior gluteal nerve)	Anterior superior iliac spine and iliac crest	Iliotibial tract	Abducts, medially rotates, and tenses iliotibial tract
Quadriceps femoris (femoral nerve)			
Rectus femoris	Anterior inferior iliac spine, ilium above acetabulum	Quadriceps tendon into base of patella, then patellar ligament onto tibia	Extends leg at knee joint; flexes hip joint
Vastus lateralis	Lateral lip of linea aspera	Same as above	Extends leg at knee joint
Vastus medialis	Medial lip of linea aspera	Same as above	Extends leg at knee joint
Vastus intermedius	Anterior, lateral, and posterior femoral shaft, from medial to lateral lip of liniea aspera	Same as above	Extends leg at knee joint
Sartorius (femoral nerve)	Anterior superior iliac spine	Superior medial surface of tibia	Flexes, abducts, and laterally rotates thigh at hip joint; flexes leg at knee joint
Psoas major (lumbar plexus, L1–L3 nerves)	T12 body, transverse processes, bodies, and intervertebral discs L1–L5	Lesser trochanter of femur	Flexes thigh on trunk
Iliacus (femoral nerve)	Ala of sacrum, iliac fossa and crest	Lesser trochanter of femur	Flexes thigh on trunk
Pectineus (femoral nerve)	Superior ramus of pubis	Pectineal line of femur inferior to lesser trochanter	Flexes and adducts thigh

Fig. 7.11 Muscles of the anterior compartment of the thigh.

The arrangement of the structures that pass under the inguinal ligament in the vascular compartment can be remembered as **NAVEL**: **N**erve (femoral branch of the genitofemoral nerve), **A**rtery, **V**ein, **E**mpty space (femoral canal), and **L**acunar ligament.

Femoral canal

The femoral canal lies within the femoral sheath, medial to the femoral vein and artery, and contains efferent lymphatics passing from the deep inguinal nodes to the abdomen (see Fig. 7.12). It provides space for expansion of the femoral vein during times of increased venous return from the lower limb. Its boundaries are the medial part of the inguinal ligament posteriorly, the lacunar ligament medially, and the femoral vein laterally.

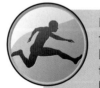

Distinguishing a femoral hernia from an indirect inguinal hernia can be difficult. Locate the pubic tubercle. If the hernial sac is superior and medial to the tubercle it is an indirect inguinal hernia; if inferior and lateral to the tubercle it is a femoral hernia.

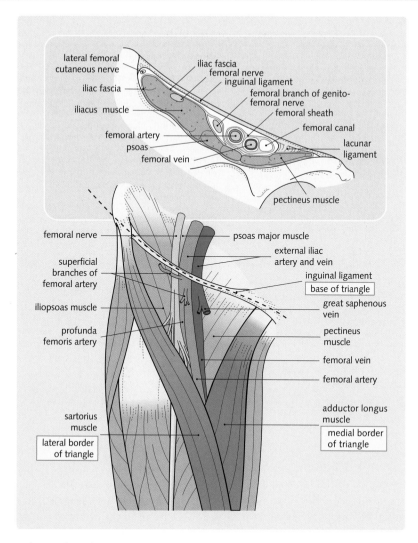

Fig. 7.12 Femoral triangle and its contents.

Adductor canal

At the apex of the femoral triangle, the femoral vessels disappear beneath the sartorius and follow the direction of the muscle to a hiatus in the tendon of the adductor magnus through which the femoral vessels reach the popliteal fossa—the adductor canal. Its contents are the femoral artery and vein, the saphenous nerve, and the nerve to the vastus medialis.

It is bounded anteriorly and laterally by the vastus medialis, posteriorly by the adductor longus and adductor magnus, and medially by the sartorius.

The femoral pulse can be palpated at the midinguinal point, halfway between the anterior superior iliac spine and the pubic symphysis.

Vessels of the thigh

Fig. 7.13 outlines the arterial supply of the thigh.

Cruciate anastomosis

The cruciate anastomosis can provide an alternative circulation should the femoral artery be obstructed.

145

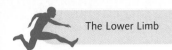

Arterial supply to the thigh		
Artery	**Origin**	**Course and distribution**
Femoral	Continuation of external iliac artery distal to inguinal ligament	Descends through femoral triangle, enters the adductor canal, and ends by passing through the adductor hiatus; supplies anterior and anteromedial surfaces of thigh
Profunda femoris	Femoral artery, 4 cm below inguinal ligament	Passes inferiorly, deep to adductus longus, to supply posterior and lateral anterior compartments of thigh
Lateral circumflex femoral	Profunda femoris; may arise from femoral artery	Passes laterally deep to sartorius and rectus femoris with an anterior branch to gluteal region, a transverse branch to the femoral neck, and a descending branch to the knee joint
Medial circumflex femoral	Profunda femoris; may arise from femoral artery	Passes medially and posteriorly between pectineus and iliopsoas and enters gluteal region; ascending and transverse branches supply the head and neck of the femur
Obturator	Internal iliac artery	Passes through obturator foramen and enters medial compartment of thigh; divides into an anterior branch to supply the obturator externus, pectineus, adductors of the thigh, and gracilis and a posterior branch to supply muscles attached to the ischial tuberosity and head of the femur

Fig. 7.13 Arterial supply to the thigh.

It is made up of:
- The inferior gluteal branch of the internal iliac artery.
- The medial and lateral circumflex femoral arteries.
- The first perforating artery from the deep femoral artery (profunda femoris).

All the perforating arteries anastomose with each other.

An accessory obturator artery arises from the inferior epigastric artery in 20% of individuals. Surgeons need to be aware of this as it is closely related to the free margin of the lacunar ligament, which is cut to release a femoral hernia.

Femoral vein
The femoral vein lies posterior to the artery in the adductor canal. Below the inguinal ligament the vein lies medial to the artery in the femoral sheath. It passes behind the inguinal ligament to become the external iliac vein.

It receives the great saphenous vein and tributaries corresponding to branches of the femoral and profunda femoris arteries.

Nerves of the thigh
The nerves of the thigh region are outlined in Fig. 7.14.

Adductor compartment of the thigh
The muscles of the adductor compartment are outlined in Fig. 7.15. They are all supplied by the obturator nerve except for the part of the adductor magnus muscle that belongs to the posterior compartment, which is supplied by the tibial division of the sciatic nerve.

The perforating branches of the profunda femoris artery and the muscular branches of the

Nerves of the thigh	
Nerve (origin)	**Course and distribution**
Ilioinguinal (lumbar plexus—L1)	Supplies skin over femoral triangle
Genitofemoral (lumbar plexus—L1–L2)	Descends on anterior surface of psoas major and divides into genital and femoral branches: femoral branch supplies skin over femoral triangle; genital branch supplies scrotum or labia majora
Lateral femoral cutaneous (lumbar plexus—L2–L3)	Passes deep to inguinal ligament, 2–3 cm medial to anterior superior iliac spine; supplies skin on anterior and lateral aspects of thigh
Anterior femoral cutaneous (femoral nerve)	Arise in femoral triangle and pierce fascia lata of thigh; supply skin on medial and anterior aspects of thigh
Posterior femoral cutaneous (sacral plexus—S1–S3)	Passes through greater sciatic foramen below piriformis; supplies skin over posterior aspect of thigh, buttock, and popliteal fossa
Femoral (lumbar plexus—L2–L4)	Passes deep to inguinal ligament in muscular compartment; supplies anterior thigh muscles, hip and knee joints, and skin on anteromedial side of thigh
Obturator (lumbar plexus—L2–L4)	Enters thigh through obturator foramen and divides: anterior branch supplies adductor longus, adductus brevis, gracilis, and pectineus; posterior branch supplies obturator externus and adductor magnus
Sciatic (sacral plexus—L4–S3)	Enters gluteal region through greater sciatic foramen below or through piriformis, descends along posterior aspect of thigh, and divides proximal to the knee into tibial and common fibular nerves; innervates hamstrings by its tibial division (except for short head of biceps femoris—innervated by common fibular division) and has articular branches to hip and knee joints

Fig. 7.14 Nerves of the thigh.

femoral artery provide the majority of the blood supply to the adductor compartment. The obturator artery also contributes proximally to the blood supply of this region.

Posterior compartment of the thigh
The muscles of the posterior compartment are outlined in Fig. 7.16 and illustrated in Fig. 7.17. They are all supplied by the tibial division of the sciatic nerve, except for the short head of the biceps (see Fig. 7.14).

Blood supply to the posterior compartment is mainly from the perforating branches of the profunda femoris, with a small contribution from the inferior gluteal artery.

Hip joint
The hip joint is a multiaxial ball-and-socket synovial joint in which the acetabulum is the socket and the head of the femur is the ball. It is a very stable joint (unlike the shoulder joint), and it supports a wide range of motion.

Stability is mainly achieved from the close fit between the femoral head and the acetabulum because more than half of the head fits within the acetabulum and acetabular labrum. Great mobility is achieved because the femoral neck is much narrower than the diameter of the head so that considerable movement may occur in all directions before the neck impinges on the acetabular labrum.

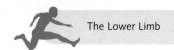

Muscles of the adductor compartment of the thigh

Name of muscle (nerve supply)	Origin	Insertion	Action
Adductor brevis (obturator nerve)	Body and inferior ramus of pubis	Pectineal line and proximal linea aspera on posterior surface of femur	Adducts thigh at hip joint
Adductor longus (obturator nerve)	Body of pubis below pubic crest	Middle third of linea aspera on posterior surface of femur	Adducts thigh at hip joint
Adductor magnus Adductor part (obturator nerve)	Ischiopubic ramus	Linea aspera on posterior surface of femur	Adducts thigh at hip joint
Hamstring part (sciatic nerve)	Ischial tuberosity	Adductor tubercle of femur	Extends thigh at hip joint
Gracilis (obturator nerve)	Body and inferior ramus of the pubis	Superior medial surface of tibia	Adducts thigh at hip joint and helps rotate thigh medially; flexes leg at knee joint
Obturator externus (obturator nerve)	Outer surface of obturator membrane, margin of obturator foramen	Trochanteric fossa	Laterally rotates thigh at hip joint

Fig. 7.15 Muscles of the adductor compartment of the thigh.

Muscles of the posterior compartment of the thigh

Name of muscle (nerve supply)	Origin	Insertion	Action
Biceps femoris Long head (common fibular division of sciatic) Short head (tibial division of sciatic)	Ischial tuberosity Linea aspera	Lateral side of head of fibula (both heads)	Flexes leg at knee joint; extends trunk when thigh and knee are flexed
Semitendinous (tibial division of sciatic)	Ischial tuberosity	Medial surface of superior part of tibial shaft	Flexes leg at knee joint; extends trunk when thigh and knee are flexed
Semimembranous (tibial division of sciatic)	Ischial tuberosity	Posterior surface of medial condyle of of the tibia; forms the oblique popliteal ligament	Flexes leg at knee joint and extends thigh at hip joint

Fig. 7.16 Muscles of the posterior compartment of the thigh.

The articular surface of the acetabulum is covered by hyaline cartilage, and it is deepened by a rim of fibrocartilage—the acetabular labrum. The labrum attaches to the transverse acetabular ligament, which crosses the acetabular notch.

The articular surface of the head of the femur is also covered by hyaline cartilage, except for a pit (fovea) where the ligament of the head of the femur attaches to the acetabulum and transverse acetabular ligament proximally and distally to the neck

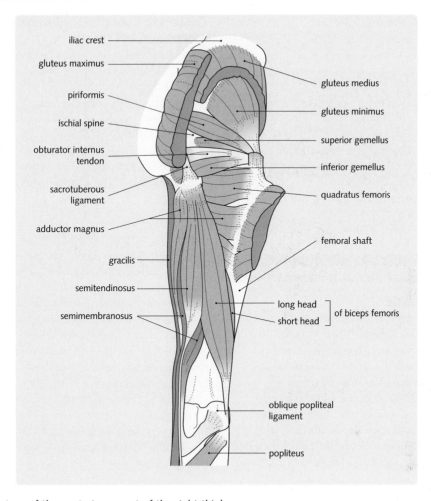

Fig. 7.17 Structure of the posterior aspect of the right thigh.

of the femur, proximal to the intertrochanteric crest.

The capsule is attached around the labrum and transverse ligament and the neck of the femur. Over the femoral neck the capsule is thrown into folds called retinacula. It is loose and strong, and a synovial membrane lines its internal surface.

The capsule is reinforced by three strong ligaments that extend from the coxal bone to the femur:

- The pubofemoral ligament from the obturator crest—prevents excessive abduction.
- The ischiofemoral ligament from the acetabular rim—prevents hyperextension.

- The iliofemoral ligament from the anterior superior iliac spine and acetabular rim—prevents hyperextension.

Blood supply is mainly from branches of the following:

- The medial circumflex femoral artery.
- The lateral circumflex femoral artery.
- The artery to the head of the femur from the obturator artery.

Nerve supply comprises the following:

- The femoral nerve.
- The superior gluteal nerve.
- The nerve to the quadratus femoris.
- The obturator nerve.

149

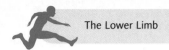

Movements of the hip joint

These are summarized in Fig. 7.18.

A femoral neck fracture is more common in people over 60, especially in women with osteoporosis. This fracture frequently tears the lateral circumflex femoral artery, which is the main blood supply to the femoral head and neck, resulting in avascular necrosis of the head.

The knee and popliteal fossa

Popliteal fossa

The diamond-shaped popliteal fossa is bordered by the biceps femoris superiorly and laterally, by the semitendinosus and semimembranosus muscles superiorly and medially, and by the lateral and medial heads of the gastrocnemius muscle inferiorly (Fig. 7.19). It is roofed by the deep fascia, which is pierced by the small saphenous vein and lymphatics. The floor is formed by the popliteal surface of the femur, the oblique popliteal ligament, and the popliteus muscle.

Contents of the popliteal fossa
Popliteus muscle (floor)

This has the following characteristics:

- Origin—a pit just below the lateral epicondyle of the femur and the lateral meniscus of the knee joint. It is intracapsular.
- Insertion—popliteal surface of the tibia, superior to the soleal line.
- Nerve supply—tibial nerve.
- Action—rotates the femur laterally on the tibia to unlock the knee and weakly flexes the knee.

Popliteal artery

This is the continuation of the femoral artery after it passes through the adductor hiatus. It terminates at the lower border of popliteus, where it divides into the anterior and posterior tibial arteries.

It gives off medial and lateral superior, middle, and medial and lateral inferior genicular arteries and muscular branches. Anastomoses of the genicular vessels with the descending genicular branch of the femoral and the descending branch of the lateral circumflex femoral and with the anterior tibial recurrent branch of the anterior tibial artery form an important collateral supply around the knee if the main vessels become occluded.

Movements at the hip joint and the muscles responsible for these movements		
Movement	Muscles involved	Factors limiting movement
Flexion	Iliopsoas, tensor fasciae latae, pectineus, sartorius, gracilis, and adductor longus, brevis, and magnus	Thigh touching abdomen, hamstring muscle tension if leg is extended
Extension	Gluteus maximus, hamstrings, adductor magnus	Iliofemoral ligament, ischiofemoral ligament
Abduction	Gluteus medius, gluteus minimus	Adductor muscle tension, pubofemoral ligament
Adduction	Adductors, gracilis, pectineus, obturator externus	Gluteus medius, gluteus minimus, other leg
Medial rotation	Tensor fasciae latae, anterior fibers of gluteus medius and gluteus minimus	Ischiofemoral ligament, iliofemoral ligament
Lateral rotation	Obturator internus, obturator externus, piriformis, gemelli, quadratus femoris, gluteus maximus	Contact of neck of femur with rim of acetabulum

Fig. 7.18 Movements at the hip joint and the muscles responsible for these movements.

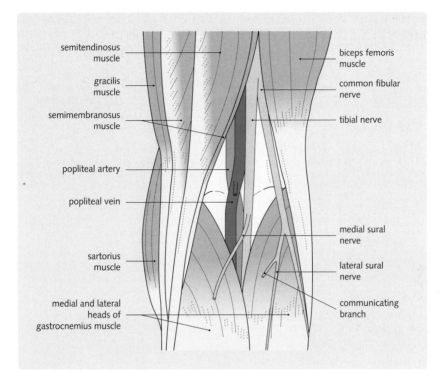

Fig. 7.19 Popliteal fossa and its contents.

Popliteal vein

This forms at the lower border of the popliteus muscle in the popliteal fossa medial to, and then ascends superficial to, the artery before entering the adductor hiatus. It receives the small saphenous vein together with veins corresponding to the arterial branches.

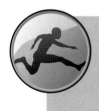

The popliteal artery is adjacent to the distal end of the femur. In fractures of the distal femur, the popliteal artery may be damaged causing it to hemorrhage.

Common fibular nerve

This lies beneath the biceps femoris in the medial border of the popliteal fossa until it reaches the head of the fibula. Branches in the popliteal fossa include:

- The lateral sural nerve, which may or may not join the medial sural nerve to supply the skin of the calf.

- A communicating branch to the medial sural nerve.
- Branches to the knee joint.

Tibial nerve

This bisects the popliteal fossa vertically. Branches in the fossa include:

- Articular branches to the knee.
- Muscular branches to soleus, gastrocnemius, plantaris, and popliteus.
- The medial sural cutaneous nerve, which joins the communicating branch of the lateral sural cutaneous nerve or a communicating branch of this nerve to form the sural nerve. The sural nerve supplies the lateral side of the leg and ankle.

Skeleton of the knee

The main features of the skeleton around the knee are illustrated in Fig. 7.20.

Knee joint

The knee joint is an articulation between the femur and the tibia, with the patella articulating with the femur anteriorly. It is a hinge type of synovial joint.

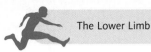

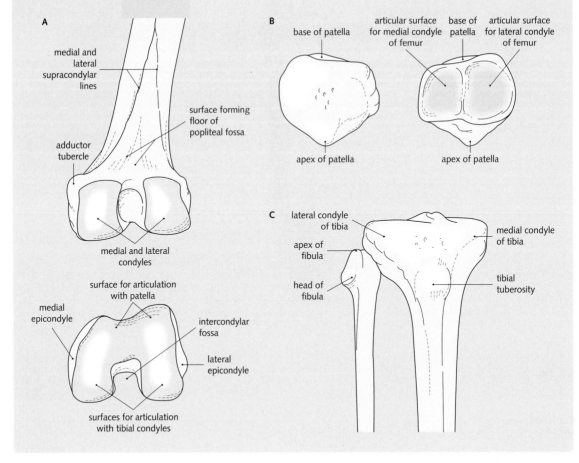

Fig. 7.20 Skeleton of the knee. (A) Posterior and inferior aspects of the lower end of right femur. (B) Anterior and posterior aspects of patella. (C) Anterior aspect of the upper end of right tibia and fibula.

The articular surfaces are covered by hyaline cartilage and consist of the margins of the femoral condyles, the patella, and the superior surface of the tibial condyles.

Capsule

This thin capsule surrounds the articular surfaces, but it is not complete. It is deficient over the lateral femoral condyle; posteroinferiorly, to allow the exit of the popliteus tendon; and anteriorly where it is replaced by the articular surface of the patella.

The capsule is strengthened anteriorly by the patellar ligament and the patellar retinacula—expansions of the tendons of the vastus medialis and lateralis that blend with the patellar ligament anteriorly. It is also reinforced by the fibular

collateral, tibial collateral, oblique popliteal, and arcuate popliteal ligaments.

Synovial membrane

The synovial membrane lines the capsule and is attached to the periphery of the patella and the edges of the menisci (Fig. 7.21). Above the patella it becomes continuous with the lining of the suprapatellar bursa. The cruciate ligaments and popliteus tendon lie outside the synovial cavity.

Ligaments

Ligaments play a major role in stabilizing the knee joint (Fig. 7.22). The cruciate ligaments keep the articular surfaces proximate to each other during the range of movement.

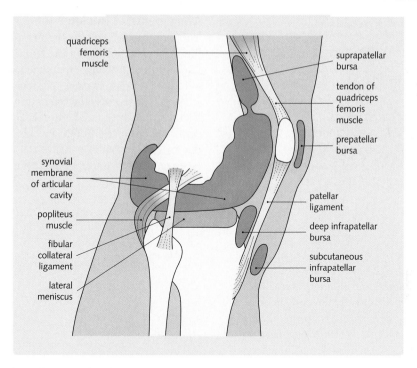

Fig. 7.21 Synovial membrane and its ligaments.

Ligaments of the knee joint	
Ligament	**Attachment**
Patellar (often called patellar tendon)	A thick fibrous band that is an extension of the quadriceps tendon, running from the patella to the tibial tuberosity; its tension is controlled by the quadriceps muscle, which stabilizes the joint through its full range of movement
Tibial or medial collateral	A flat, strong band from the medial femoral epicondyle to the tibia
Fibular or lateral collateral	A rounded, cord-like band from the superior medial surface of the lateral femoral condyle to the fibular head
Oblique popliteal	Expansion of the semimembranous tendon, which reniforces the capsule posteriorly
Anterior cruciate	From the anterior part of the intercondylar area of the tibia to the medial surface of the lateral femoral condyle
Posterior cruciate	From the posterior part of the intercondylar area of the tibia to the lateral surface of the medial femoral condyle
Arcuate popliteal	The thickened edge of the joint capsule where it arches over the exiting popliteus muscle

Fig. 7.22 Ligaments of the knee joint.

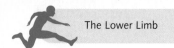

Inflammation of the knee joint cavity can spread to the suprapatellar bursa through its communication. The resulting increase in synovial fluid due to inflammation can, therefore, be palpated and aspirated from this bursa.

Movements at the knee joint

The movements at the knee joint are outlined in Fig. 7.24. The 'locking of the knee joint' puts the knee into a slightly hyperextended position, and the joint is an extremely stable platform for the femur.

As the knee extends, the anterior cruciate ligament becomes taut, preventing posterior displacement of the femur on the tibia. However, due to a larger surface area of the medial condyle (see Fig. 7.20), passive medial rotation of the

Menisci

The menisci are two crescentic plates of fibrocartilage (Fig. 7.23), which are thicker at their external margins and thinner internally. The menisci are attached to the intercondylar area of the tibia and at the periphery to the fibrous capsule. A fibrous band, the transverse ligament of the knee, joins their anterior edges. They deepen the articular surfaces of the tibia and act as shock absorbers.

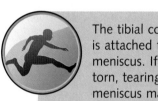

The tibial collateral ligament is attached to the medial meniscus. If this ligament is torn, tearing of the medial meniscus may also occur.

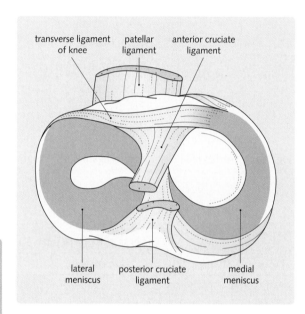

Fig. 7.23 Menisci and their ligaments, viewed from above.

Movements at the knee joint	
Movement	**Muscle**
Flexion	Hamstrings, gastrocnemius, gracilis
Extension	Quadriceps femoris
Medial and lateral rotation of flexed knee	Hamstrings
Unlocking of knee	Popliteus
Locking of knee—a passive medial rotation of the femur on the tibia	Occurs at the end of extension by the anterior cruciate ligament becoming taut and the femoral medidal condyle moving round the ligament

Fig. 7.24 Movements at the knee joint.

femur occurs on the tibia, which tightens the collateral ligaments. At the end of this movement the knee becomes locked.

The knee joint must be unlocked before flexion can occur. This is performed by the popliteus muscle, which laterally rotates the femur, relaxing the ligaments sufficiently to allow flexion.

Blood and nerve supply of the knee joint
Blood supply comes from the genicular branches of the popliteal artery.

Nerve supply comprises the articular branches of the sciatic, femoral, and obturator nerves.

Bursae around the knee joint
There are more than 12 bursae around the knee joint. The main ones are (see Fig. 7.21):
- The suprapatellar bursa, which is continuous with the joint cavity.
- The prepatellar bursa, which is subcutaneous.
- The superficial infrapatellar bursa, which is also subcutaneous.
- The deep infrapatellar bursa, beneath the patellar ligament.

The leg and foot

Skeleton of the leg
Important features of the bones of the leg are illustrated in Fig. 7.25.

The interosseous membrane is a tough band of tissue linking the interosseous borders of the tibia and fibula. It has a large oval opening near its proximal end, through which pass the anterior tibial vessels. Inferiorly it is pierced by a branch of the fibular artery.

Proximal tibiofibular joint
This is a plane type of synovial joint between the head of the fibular and the lateral tibial condyle. It is surrounded by a fibrous capsule that is reinforced by the anterior and posterior tibiofibular ligaments and the anterior and posterior ligaments of the head of the fibula, which tie the head to the lateral tibial condyle.

Inferior tibiofibular joint
The inferior tibiofibular joint is an articulation between the lower end of the tibia and fibula. It is a fibrous joint stabilized by the interosseus ligament

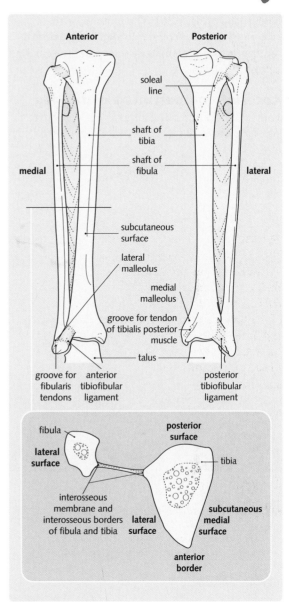

Fig. 7.25 Anterior and posterior features of the right tibia and fibula, and the relationship of the two bones and the interosseous membrane in cross-section.

and the anterior and posterior inferior tibiofibular ligaments. It allows little movement, and it stabilizes the ankle joint by keeping the lateral malleolus firmly against the lateral surface of the talus.

Compartments of the leg
The leg is divided into anterior, posterior, and lateral compartments by septa from the crural

155

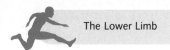

(deep) fascia (Fig. 7.26). The muscles of the posterior compartment are divided into superficial and deep groups by the transverse intermuscular septum.

Anterior compartment of the leg
Muscles of the anterior compartment are shown in Figs 7.27 and 7.28.

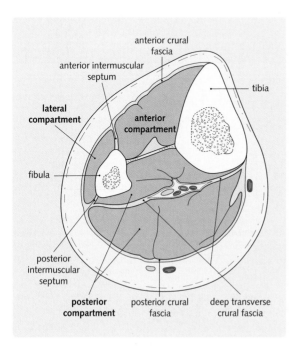

Fig. 7.26 Compartments of the leg.

Vessels of the anterior compartment
The anterior tibial artery is the vessel of the anterior compartment (Figs 7.29 and 7.30). It is a terminal branch of the popliteal artery.

Nerves of the anterior compartment
The common fibular nerve (L4–L5, S1–S2) leaves the popliteal fossa to enter the lateral compartment of the leg by winding around the neck of the fibula (Fig. 7.31). Here, it divides into the superficial and deep fibular nerves. The deep fibular nerve passes through the extensor digitorum longus into the anterior compartment.

The common fibular nerve is vulnerable to injury, e.g., by a car bumper, as it passes around the fibula. Damage results in footdrop.

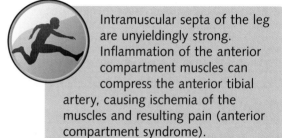
Intramuscular septa of the leg are unyieldingly strong. Inflammation of the anterior compartment muscles can compress the anterior tibial artery, causing ischemia of the muscles and resulting pain (anterior compartment syndrome).

Muscles of the anterior compartment of the leg			
Name of muscle (nerve supply)	**Origin**	**Insertion**	**Action**
Extensor digitorum longus (deep fibular nerve)	Fibula and interosseus membrane	Extensor expansion of lateral four toes	Extends toes and dorsiflexes foot at ankle joint
Extensor hallucis longus (deep fibular nerve)	Fibula and interosseus membrane	Base of distal phalanx of great toe	Extends big toe and dorsiflexes foot at ankle joint
Fibularis tertius (deep fibular nerve)	Fibula and interosseus membrane	Base of 5th metatarsal bone	Dorsiflexes and everts foot
Tibialis anterior (deep fibular nerve)	Tibia and interosseus membrane	Medial cuneiform and base of 1st metatarsal bone	Dorsiflexes and inverts foot

Fig. 7.27 Muscles of the anterior compartment of the leg.

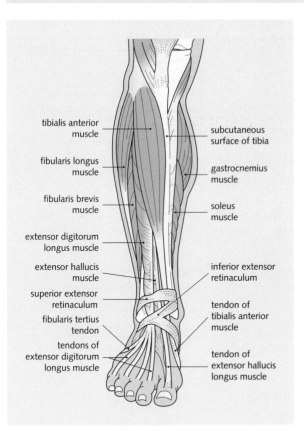

Fig. 7.28 Extensor muscles of the anterior compartment of the leg.

tibialis anterior muscle

subcutaneous surface of tibia

fibularis longus muscle

gastrocnemius muscle

fibularis brevis muscle

soleus muscle

extensor digitorum longus muscle

extensor hallucis muscle

inferior extensor retinaculum

superior extensor retinaculum

tendon of tibialis anterior muscle

fibularis tertius tendon

tendons of extensor digitorum longus muscle

tendon of extensor hallucis longus muscle

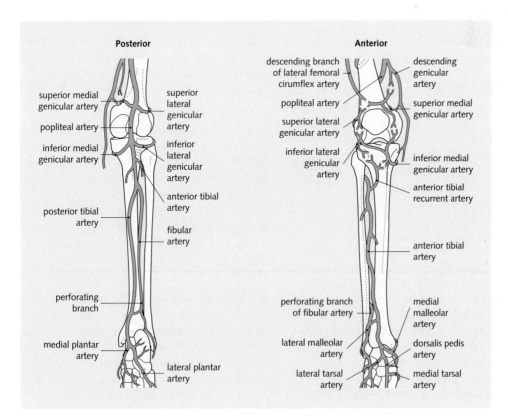

Posterior

Anterior

superior medial genicular artery

superior lateral genicular artery

popliteal artery

inferior medial genicular artery

inferior lateral genicular artery

anterior tibial artery

posterior tibial artery

fibular artery

perforating branch

medial plantar artery

lateral plantar artery

descending branch of lateral femoral cirumflex artery

descending genicular artery

popliteal artery

superior medial genicular artery

superior lateral genicular artery

inferior lateral genicular artery

inferior medial genicular artery

anterior tibial recurrent artery

anterior tibial artery

perforating branch of fibular artery

medial malleolar artery

lateral malleolar artery

dorsalis pedis artery

lateral tarsal artery

medial tarsal artery

Fig. 7.29 Arterial supply to the posterior and anterior compartments of the leg.

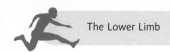

Arterial supply to the leg		
Artery (origin)	**Course**	**Distribution**
Popliteal (continuation of femoral artery at adductor hiatus)	Passes through popliteal fossa to leg; ends at lower border of popliteal muscle by dividing into anterior and posterior tibial arteries	Medial and lateral superior, middle, and medial and lateral inferior genicular arteries to both internal and medial aspects of knee
Anterior tibial (popliteal artery)	Passes into anterior compartment through gap in superior part of interosseus membrane and descends on the membrane between the tibialis anterior and extensor digitorum longus muscles	Anterior compartment of the leg
Dorsal pedis (continuation of anterior tibial artery distal to inferior extensor retinaculum)	Runs on the dorsum of the foot and gives rise to tarsal, arcuate, and dorsal metatarsal arteries; descends through the first interosseus space to join plantar arch	Muscles on dorsum of foot; pierces first dorsal interosseus muscle to contribute to formation of plantar arch
Posterior tibial (popliteal artery)	Passes through posterior compartment of leg and terminates distal to flexor retinaculum by dividing into medial and lateral plantar arteries	Posterior and lateral compartments of leg; nutrient artery passes to tibia; circumflex fibular branch contributes to knee anastomoses
Fibular (posterior tibial artery)	Descends in posterior compartment adjacent to posterior gastrocnemius septum	Posterior compartment of leg; perforating branches supply lateral compartment of leg

Fig. 7.30 Arterial supply to the leg.

Dorsum of the foot

The structures from the anterior compartment pass onto the dorsum of the foot. The extensor digitorum longus becomes tendinous proximal to the ankle and continues as the lateral four digits of the foot to join an extensor expansion. These expansions have the same arrangement as those found in the medial four digits of the hand. Over the proximal phalanx each expansion splits into three slips. A central slip inserts into the middle phalanx. Two lateral slips converge into the distal phalanx. The dorsal and plantar interossei and lumbrical muscles insert into each expansion.

The extensor digitorum brevis and extensor hallucis brevis muscles are the only muscles intrinsic to the dorsum of the foot. The tendon of the extensor hallucis longus passes onto the dorsum of the foot medial to the extensor digitorum longus tendons on its way to the distal phalanx of the big toe. Arising from the superolateral surface of the calcaneus, the three tendons of extensor digitorum brevis join the lateral sides of the extensor digitorum longus tendons for the middle three toes over the metatarsophalangeal joint. From a similar origin,

the extensor hallucis brevis tendon inserts into the base of the proximal phalanx of the hallux (great toe). The muscle belly of this tendon is usually separate from the rest of the muscle. The nerve supply is by the deep fibular nerve and both muscles assist in extending the digits (toes).

Extensor retinacula

The superior and inferior extensor retinacula keep the extensor tendons firmly bound down to the dorsum of the foot (Fig. 7.32). The retinacula are deep fascia that is an extension of the anterior crural fascia.

The superior band passes from the anterior border of the tibia to the anterior border of the fibula. The inferior band is Y-shaped, and it runs from the calcaneus to the medial malleolus and plantar fascia.

Nerves and vessels of the dorsum of the foot

The deep fibular nerve and anterior tibial artery enter the foot beneath the extensor retinacula between the tendons of the extensor digitorum longus and the extensor hallucis longus. The anterior tibial artery continues as the dorsalis pedis artery at the ankle joint (see Fig. 7.30).

Nerves of the leg	
Nerve (origin)	**Course and distribution**
Common fibular (sciatic nerve)	Arises at apex of popliteal fossa and follows medial border of biceps femoris and its tendon; passes over posterior aspect of head of fibula and then winds around neck of fibula, deep to fibularis longus, where it divides into deep and superficial fibular neves; supplies skin on posterolateral part of leg via its branch, lateral sural cutaneous nerve
Deep fibular (common fibular nerve)	Arises between fibularis longus and neck of fibula; descends on interosseus membrane and enters dorsum of foot, supplies anterior muscles of leg and skin of first interdigital web
Saphenous (femoral nerve)	Arises in the femoral triangle, emerges from the adductor canal on the medial side of the knee to descend with the great saphenous vein; supplies skin on medial side of leg and foot
Superficial fibular (common fibular nerve)	Arises between fibularis longus and neck of fibula and descends in lateral compartment of leg; supplies peroneus longus and brevis and skin on anterior surface of leg; pierces deep fascia of distal leg to supply dorsum of foot
Tibial (sciatic nerve)	Descends through popliteal fossa and lies on popliteus; then runs inferiorly with posterior tibial vessels and terminates beneath flexor retinaculum by dividing into medial and lateral plantar nerves; supplies posterior muscles of leg, knee joint, and skin and muscles of the sole of the foot

Fig. 7.31 Nerves of the leg.

The dorsalis pedis artery can be palpated between the extensor hallucis longus tendon and the extensor digitorum longus tendon, on top of the navicular bone. A diminished or absent pulse may indicate peripheral vascular disease.

Contraction of the superficial calf muscles (triceps surae) acts as a venous pump, pushing the blood superiorly. The deep fascia improves the pumping action by acting as an elastic stocking.

Lateral compartment of the leg

The contents of the lateral compartment are shown in Fig. 7.33. Its muscles are outlined in Fig. 7.34.

Posterior compartment of the leg

Fig. 7.35 outlines the muscles of the posterior compartment.

For the structures passing behind the medial malleolus remember the mnemonic: **T**om, **D**ick **A**nd **V**ery **N**aughty **H**arry (**t**ibialis posterior, flexor **d**igitorum longus, **a**rtery, **v**ein, **n**erve, flexor **h**allucis longus).

159

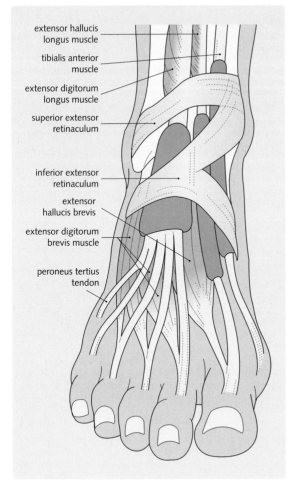

Fig. 7.32 Structures of the extensor retinacula.

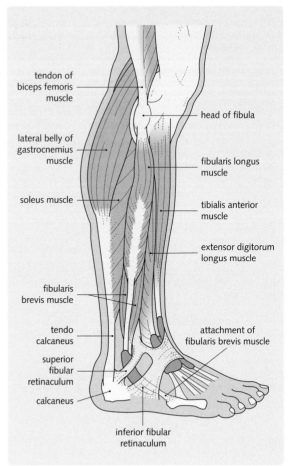

Fig. 7.33 Lateral compartment of the leg and its structures.

Muscles of the lateral compartment of the leg			
Name of muscle (nerve supply)	Origin	Insertion	Action
Fibularis longus (superficial fibular nerve)	Head and superior lateral surface of fibula	Base of 1st metatarsal and medial cuneiform	Everts and weakly plantarflexes the foot
Fibularis brevis (superficial fibular nerve)	Inferior lateral surface of fibula	Dorsal surface of tuberosity of 5th metatarsal bone	Everts and weakly plantarflexes the foot

Fig. 7.34 Muscles of the lateral compartment of the leg.

Muscles of the posterior compartment of the leg			
Name of muscle (nerve supply)	Origin	Insertion	Action
Superficial group			
Plantaris (tibial nerve)	Lateral supracondyle ridge of femur	Via tendo calcaneus (Achilles tendon) into posterior surface of calcaneus	Plantarflexes foot at ankle joint
Soleus (tibial nerve)	Medial border of posterior tibia	Via tendo calcaneus (Achilles tendon) into posterior surface of calcaneus	Plantarflexes foot at ankle joint
Gastrocnemius (tibial nerve)	Medial surface of lateral condyle and surface of femur superior to medial condyle	Via tendo calcaneus (Achilles tendon) into posterior surface of calcaneus	Plantarflexes foot at ankle joint; raises heel during walking; flexes leg at knee joint
Deep group			
Flexor digitorum longus (tibial nerve)	Posterior tibia inferior to soleal line	Bases of distal phalanges of lateral four toes	Flexes lateral four toes; plantarflexes foot
Flexor hallucis longus (tibial nerve)	Inferior two-thirds of of posterior fibula, interosseus membrane	Base of distal phalanx of big toe	Flexes big toe; weakly plantarflexes foot
Tibialis posterior (tibial nerve)	Posterior tibia inferior to soleal line, posterior fibula, and interosseus membrane	Tuberosity of navicular bone and cuneiform and cuboid bones and bases of 2–4 metatarsals	Planterflexes and inverts foot

Fig. 7.35 Muscles of the posterior compartment of the leg.

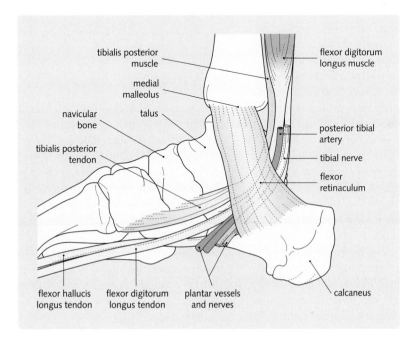

Fig. 7.36 Flexor retinaculum.

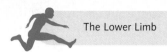

Flexor retinaculum

The flexor retinaculum runs from the medial
malleolus to the calcaneus and plantar fascia (Fig.
7.36). The deep flexor muscles are also surrounded
for a short distance by tendon sheaths.

The space beneath the retinaculum is divided by
three septa into four compartments. Occupying
these compartments, from anterior to posterior, are:
- The tendon of the tibialis posterior.
- The tendon of the flexor digitorum longus.
- The tibial nerve and posterior tibial vessels.
- The tendon of the flexor hallucis longus.

Skeleton of the foot

The skeleton of the foot consists of the tarsal
bones, the metatarsal bones, and the phalanges
(Fig. 7.37).

The body weight is transferred to the talus
from the tibia, then posteriorly to the calcaneus,
and anteriorly to the heads of the 2nd–5th
metatarsals and sesamoid bones of the 1st digit.
The metatarsal bones are composed of a base
proximally, a body, and a distal head. The first
digit (the hallux) has two phalanges; the others
have three (proximal, middle, and distal).

Ankle joint

The ankle joint is a hinge type of joint between the
superior surface of the talus and the distal ends of
the tibia and fibula, including the medial and lateral
malleoli.

It is a synovial joint, and it allows only flexion and
extension. Dorsiflexion (extension) involves the
tibialis anterior, extensor digitorum longus, and
extensor hallucis longus. Plantarflexion (flexion)
involves gastrocnemius, soleus, flexor digitorum
longus, flexor hallucis longus, and tibialis posterior.

The joint is surrounded by a capsule that is thin
anteroposteriorly and reinforced by strong medial
and lateral ligaments. The medial (deltoid)
ligament runs from the medial malleolus to
the tuberosity of the navicular bone via the
tibionavicular ligament, to the calcaneus via the
tibiocalcaneal ligament, and to the talus via
the anterior and posterior tibiotalar ligaments.
The lateral ligament arises from the lateral
malleolus, and it is attached to the neck of the
talus via the anterior talofibular ligament, to the
lateral tubercle by the tibiofibular ligament, and to
the calcaneus by the calcaneofibular ligament.

The articular surface of the talus is wedge
shaped, and has a round, superior surface that

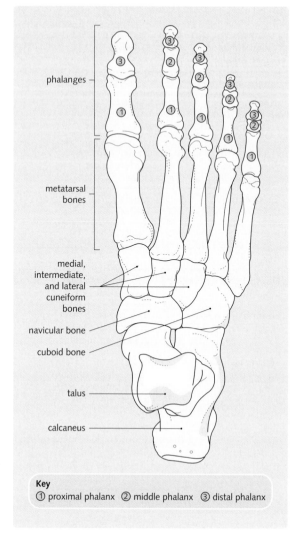

Key
① proximal phalanx ② middle phalanx ③ distal phalanx

Fig. 7.37 Skeleton of the foot.

articulates with the inferior surface of the distal
tibia, transferring weight from the tibia to the talus.
The malleoli on either side grip the talus tightly as
it rocks on its articular surface. The articular
surface is wider anteriorly than posteriorly. As a
result the ankle joint is most stable in dorsiflexion
because the wider anterior border is 'driven'
between the two malleoli, which clasp it.

The ankle is the most frequently injured joint in
the body. Ankle sprains are usually inversion
injuries since the lateral ligament is slightly weaker
than the deltoid ligament and is, therefore, usually
damaged. Severe damage to the ligament results in
an unstable joint.

Blood supply is from the fibular and anterior
and posterior tibial arteries.

Remember that the talar articular surface is wedge shaped, being wider anteriorly. Therefore, the ankle joint is most stable in dorsiflexion.

The lateral ligament of the ankle is weaker than the deltoid (medial) ligament. Therefore, a sprained ankle is almost always an inversion injury because the lateral ligament tears more commonly.

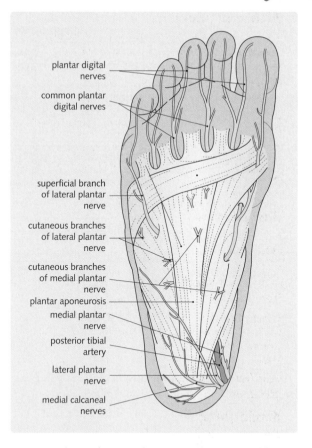

Fig. 7.38 Plantar fascia and cutaneous innervation of the sole of the foot.

Nerve supply is from the tibial and deep fibular nerves.

Sole of the foot

The sole bears the weight of the body. The skin is thick and hairless, with numerous sweat glands. Fibrous septa divide the subcutaneous fat into small loculi, and they anchor the skin to the deep fascia or plantar aponeurosis (Fig. 7.38). The fat-filled areas, particularly the heel, are shock absorbing.

The plantar aponeurosis extends from the calcaneal tuberosity and divides into five bifurcating slips that become continuous with the flexor fibrous sheaths at the base of the toes and that are reinforced there by the superficial transverse metatarsal ligaments. The bifurcation allows passage of the flexor tendons. It is very strong, protects the underlying muscles, vessels, and nerves, helps hold the parts of the foot together, and helps support the long arch of the foot. It is perforated by the cutaneous nerves supplying the sole of the foot.

The muscles of the sole of the foot are in four layers (Fig. 7.39). The axis of abduction and adduction passes through the second digit. Therefore, digits either move towards (adduction) or away (abduction) from the second digit.

Nerves of the foot

The nerves of the foot are described in Figs. 7.40 and 7.41.

Cutaneous innervation of the dorsum of the foot is mainly from the superficial fibular nerve, with the deep fibular nerve innervating the web space between the first and second digits, the sural nerve innervating the lateral side of the foot, and the saphenous nerve innervating the medial side of the foot.

Blood supply to the foot

The posterior tibial artery terminates by dividing into the medial and lateral plantar arteries beneath the flexor retinaculum (Fig. 7.42).

The medial plantar artery passes forward with the medial plantar nerve. It gives off branches to the muscles of the first digit, digital branches accompanying those of the medial plantar nerve, and terminates as a plantar digital branch to the medial side of the big toe and a branch that joins the deep plantar arch.

The lateral plantar artery crosses the sole of the foot between the quadratus plantae and flexor

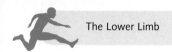

Intrinsic plantar muscles of the foot			
Muscle	Origin	Insertion	Action
First layer			
Abductor hallucis (medial plantar nerve)	Medial tubercle of calcaneus, flexor retinaculum, plantar aponeurosis	Medial side of base of proximal phalanx of hallux	Abducts and flexes hallux (big toe)
Flexor digitorum brevis (medial plantar nerve)	Medial tubercle of calcaneus, plantar aponeurosis	Each tendon bifurcates and inserts into the middle phalanx of the lateral four digits	Flexes lateral four toes
Abductor digiti minimi (lateral plantar nerve)	Medial and lateral tubercles of calcaneus, plantar aponeurosis	Lateral side of base of proximal phalanx of fifth digit	Abducts and flexes fifth digit (little toe)
Second layer			
Quadratus plantae (lateral plantar nerve)	Medial and lateral plantar surface of calcaneus	Posterolateral margin of tendon of flexor digitorum longus	Pulls on the tendon of flexor digitorum longus to assist in flexion of lateral four digits
Lumbricals (first medial lumbrical: medial plantar nerve; lateral three lumbricals: lateral plantar nerve)	Tendons of flexor digitorum longus	Medial side of extensor expansions of lateral four digits	Flex MTP joint, extend at DIP and PIP joints
Third layer			
Flexor hallucis brevis (medial plantar nerve)	Plantar surface of cuboid and lateral cuneiform	Both sides of base of proximal phalanx of hallux	Flexes proximal phalanx of hallux
Adductor hallucis (deep branch of lateral plantar nerve) Oblique head Transverse head	Second to fourth metatarsal bases and plantar ligament of MTP joints	Both heads insert into the lateral side of the base of the proximal phalanx of the hallux	Both heads abduct hallux toward second toe
Flexor digiti minimi (superficial branch of lateral plantar nerve)	Base of fifth metatarsal	Base of proximal phalanx of fifth digit	Flexes proximal phalanx of fifth digit (little toe)
Fourth layer			
Plantar interossei (lateral plantar nerve)	Bases and medial sides of the third, fourth, and fifth metatarsals	Bases of proximal phalanges of the third, fourth, and fifth digits	Abduct digits toward second digit, flex MTP joint, extend at DIP and PIP joints
Dorsal interossei (lateral plantar nerve)	Adjacent sides of first and second; second and third; third and fourth; and fourth and fifth metatarsals	Medial side of proximal phalanx of the first digit, lateral sides of proximal phalanges of second through fourth digits and their extensor expansions	Abduct digits away from second digit. With palmar interossei and lumbricals, they extend DIP and PIP joints and flex MTP joint

Fig. 7.39 Intrinsic plantar muscles of the foot (IP, interphalangeal joint; PIP, proximal interphalangeal joint; DIP, distal interphalangeal joint; MTP, metatarsophalangeal joint).

digitorum brevis, and it gives off muscular and cutaneous branches. At the level of the base of the 5th metatarsal, the artery passes medially and anastomoses with the deep dorsal plantar artery from the dorsalis pedis artery to form the plantar arch. From this arch plantar metatarsal arteries arise, which divide to form the plantar digital arteries for the toes.

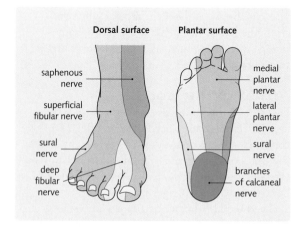

Fig. 7.40 Distribution of nerves of the foot.

Fibrous flexor and flexor synovial sheaths

As the tendons for each toe from the flexor digitorum longus and the underlying flexor digitorum brevis reach the level of the metatarsal heads, they acquire a digital fibrous sheath lined with a synovial sheath, both of which extend to the base of the distal phalanx. This arrangement is essentially similar to that in the hand. There are synovial sheaths that invest the flexor digitorum longus and flexor hallucis longus tendons from beneath the flexor retinaculum to the base of the metatarsals, but there is no continuity between these and the more distal synovial sheaths. The synovial sheath for tibialis posterior extends from the flexor retinaculum to the tendon's insertion into the navicular bone.

Intertarsal joints of the foot

The intertarsal joints of the foot occur between the articulating tarsal bones. All are synovial joints except the cuboidonavicular joint, which is a fibrous joint.

Subtalar (talocalcaneal) joint

The subtalar joint is formed by the articulation of the talus with the calcaneus posteriorly. It is

Outline of the nerves of the foot	
Nerve (origin)	**Distribution**
Saphenous (femoral nerve)	Supplies skin on medial side of foot as far anteriorly as head of first metatarsal
Superficial fibular (common fibular nerve)	Supplies skin on dorsum of foot and all digits, except adjoining sides of first and second digits and lateral side of fifth digit
Deep fibular (common fibular nerve)	Supplies extensor digitorum brevis, extensor hallucis brevis, and skin on contiguous sides of first and second digits
Medial plantar (larger terminal branch of the tibial nerve)	Supplies skin of medial side of sole of foot and sides of first three and one-half digits; also supplies abductor hallucis, flexor digitorum brevis, flexor hallucis brevis, and first lumbrical
Lateral plantar (smaller terminal branch of the tibial nerve)	Supplies quadratus plantae, abductor digiti minimi, and flexor digiti minimi brevis; deep branch supplies plantar and dorsal interossei, lateral three lumbricals, and adductor hallucis; supplies skin on sole lateral to a line splitting fourth digit
Sural (tibial and common fibular nerves)	Lateral aspect of foot and posterior and middle of the sole of foot
Calcaneal nerves (tibial and sural nerves)	Skin of heel

Fig. 7.41 Nerves of the foot.

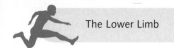

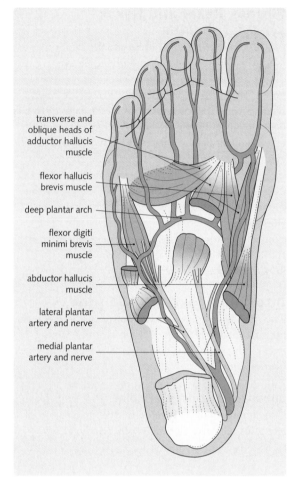

transverse and oblique heads of adductor hallucis muscle

flexor hallucis brevis muscle

deep plantar arch

flexor digiti minimi brevis muscle

abductor hallucis muscle

lateral plantar artery and nerve

medial plantar artery and nerve

Fig. 7.42 Blood and nerve supply to the sole of the foot.

strengthened by the talocalcaneal ligaments. Inversion and eversion movements of the heel occur at this joint.

Transverse tarsal joint

This is a compound joint made up of two transversely aligned intertarsal joints: the calcaneocuboid joint between the calcaneus and the cuboid bones laterally, and the more complex talocalcaneonavicular joint between the talus, navicular, and calcaneus medially. The talonavicular portion of this joint is the main contributor to the transverse tarsal joint. The talocalcaneonavicular joint is supported by the spring (calcaneonavicular) ligament. The calcaneocuboidal joint occurs between the calcaneus and cuboid bone. It is

supported mainly by the long and short plantar ligaments.

The transverse tarsal joint serves as a link between the hindfoot and midfoot, and its movements are chiefly inversion and eversion of the forefoot. Inversion and eversion movement of the heel and forefoot occur synchronously, involving both the subtalar and transverse talar joints.

Other tarsal joints

The cuneonavicular, cuboideonavicular, intercuneiform, and cuneocuboidal joints are strengthened by ligaments of the same names. Independent movement is not possible at any of these joints.

Arches of the foot

Each foot has a lateral and a medial longitudinal arch. If the feet are placed side by side, a transverse arch is considered to be present across the bases of the metatarsals. These arches support the weight of the body, and they are maintained by bone shape, muscles, and ligaments.

The medial is higher and more important than the lateral arch, and it consists of the calcaneus, talus, navicular, and cuneiform bones and the medial three metatarsals. The talus acts as a keystone in the center of the arch. The plantar calcaneonavicular (spring), long and short plantar ligaments, and the strong plantar aponeurosis maintain the longitudinal arch. The abductor and flexor muscles in the first and third layers, and the flexor digitorum longus tendon support this arch. Finally, the tibialis posterior and fibularis longus tendons suspend and stabilize the arch during stance.

The lower lateral arch consists of the calcaneus, the cuboid, and the lateral two metatarsals. This is maintained by the long and short (calcaneocuboidal) plantar ligaments, the plantar aponeurosis, the abductor and short flexor muscles, and the tibialis posterior and fibularis longus tendons.

Each foot contains half of the transverse arch. Each half consists of the metatarsal bases, cuboid, and the three cuneiforms. It is maintained by the wedge shape of the cuneiform bones and metatarsal bases, the strong long and short plantar ligaments, as well as the deep transverse metatarsal ligaments. The peroneus longus and brevis tendons suspend and tie the arch ends together.

Functions of the feet

The feet serve to:

- Support the body weight when standing.
- Maintain balance.
- Act as propulsive levers (e.g., in walking and running).

In older people, prolonged periods of standing can weaken and stretch the plantar ligaments and aponeurosis, particularly under excessive body weight. As a result the medial longitudinal arch 'falls,' causing a flat foot (pes planus). The appearance of a flat foot before the age of 3 is usually normal and resolves with age.

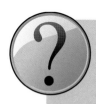

- Describe the superficial venous drainage of the lower limb.
- Outline the cutaneous innervation of the lower limb.
- Describe the lymphatic drainage of the lower limb and how this is related to venous drainage.
- Outline the skeleton of the hip and thigh region.
- What is the fascia lata?
- Describe the muscles and contents of the gluteal region.
- What are the boundaries and contents of the femoral triangle?
- Discuss the arterial supply of the thigh.
- Discuss the anatomy of the hip joint.
- Discuss the muscles of the anterior, posterior, and adductor compartments of the thigh.
- What are the boundaries and contents of the popliteal fossa?
- Outline the anatomy of the knee joint.
- Describe the arterial anastomosis around the knee.
- List the muscles of each compartment of the leg, their function, and innervation.
- Describe the arterial supply of the leg.
- Describe the nerve supply of the leg.
- Describe the skeleton of the foot.
- Describe the anatomy of the dorsum of the foot.
- Describe the anatomy of the ankle joint, including its ligaments.
- Describe the arrangement and contents of the four muscle layers of the plantar surface of the foot.
- Discuss the blood and nerve supply of the sole of the foot.
- Describe the arches of the foot and their reinforcing ligaments.
- Describe the relevant joints and reinforcing ligaments related to inversion and eversion of the foot.

8. The Head and Neck

Regions and components of the head and neck

Skull

The skull is composed of 22 bones joined at sutures or synovial joints. The bones of the skull may be divided into:
- The cranium.
- The facial skeleton.

The cranium is subdivided into:
- An upper part—the calvaria (skullcap).
- A lower part—the base of the skull.

Superior aspect of the skull

A view of the skull from above (norma verticalis) is illustrated in Fig. 8.1.

Posterior aspect of the skull

A view of the skull from behind (norma occipitalis) is shown in Fig. 8.2. Note the mastoid process of the temporal bone and the external occipital protuberance—a midline elevation from the occipital bone—from which the superior nuchal line extends laterally.

Frontal aspect of the skull

The skull is viewed from the front (norma frontalis) in Fig. 8.3. The frontal bones form the forehead and the superior margin of the orbits. They articulate with the nasal bones, intersecting at the nasion, and with the frontal processes of the maxilla (upper jaw) and zygomatic bones. The mandible (lower jaw) is a U-shaped bone that articulates with the temporal bone at the temperomandibular joint. Both mandible and maxilla support teeth.

Lateral aspect of the skull

Fig. 8.4 shows the lateral view (norma lateralis) of the skull. The parietal bone articulates with the

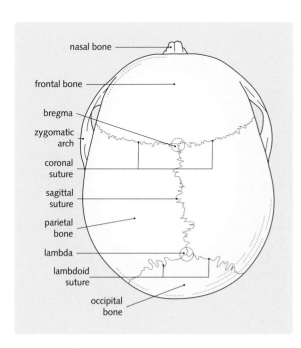

Fig. 8.1 Skull viewed from above.

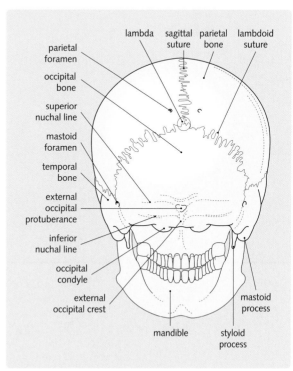

Fig. 8.2 Skull viewed from behind.

169

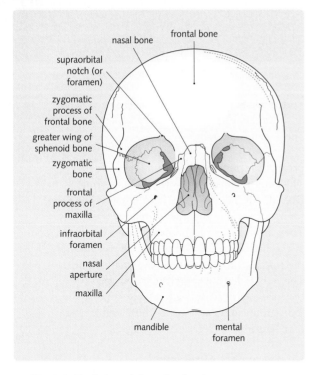

Fig. 8.3 Skull viewed from the front.

greater wing of the sphenoid bone and the temporal bone. These three bones meet at a point, the pterion, which is the thinnest part of the lateral aspect of the skull and vulnerable to damage. The middle meningeal artery lies just deep to this point, and this may rupture following trauma to the head.

The zygomatic arch is formed by the zygomatic process of the temporal bone and the temporal process of the zygomatic bone.

Trauma to the pterion can tear the middle meningeal artery and cause bleeding externally to the dura mater (epidural hemorrhage).

Basal aspect of the skull

In Fig. 8.5 the skull is viewed from below (norma basalis). The palate is formed by the palatine process of the maxilla and the horizontal processes of the palatine bones. The alveolar process of the maxilla surrounds the palate.

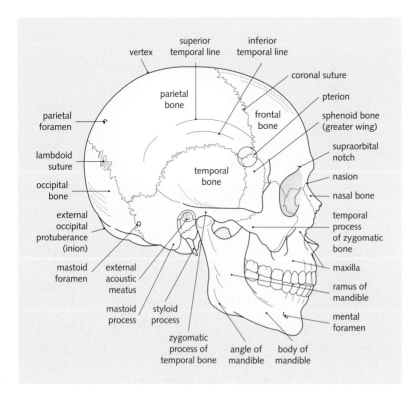

Fig. 8.4 Lateral view of the skull.

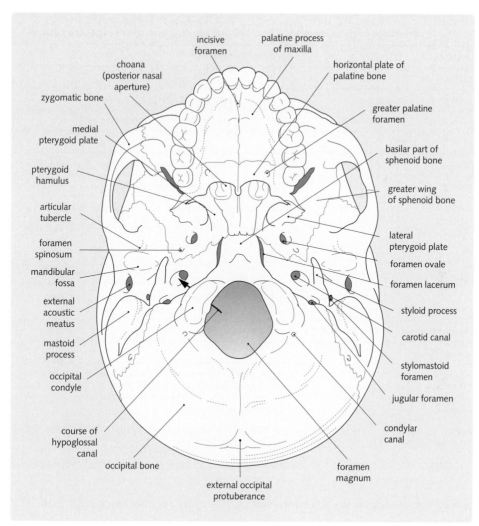

Fig. 8.5 Skull seen from below.

Openings in the skull
Fig. 8.6 lists the important openings in the base of the skull and their contents.

Cervical vertebrae
There are seven cervical vertebrae forming the skeleton of the neck. All except C1 (atlas), C2 (axis), and C7 are typical vertebrae. C7 possesses a longer spinous process, which is usually the most superior spinous process that is palpable (see Chapter 2).

The face and scalp

Scalp
The scalp consists of five layers (Fig. 8.7), and it has a very rich blood supply (Fig. 8.8). Injuries to this region often result in profuse bleeding.

The arteries of the scalp course within the connective tissue layer between the skin and the epicranial aponeurosis of the frontalis, occipitalis, temperoparietialis, and superior auricular muscles. The scalp veins follow the arterial supply:

171

The important openings in the base of the skull and the structures that pass through them	
Foramen or aperture	**Structures transmitted**
Anterior cranial fossa	
Cribiform foramina in cribiform plate	Axons of olfactory nerves
Anterior and posterior ethmoid foramina	Anterior and posterior ethmoid vessels and nerve
Middle cranial fossa	
Foramen ovale	V_3 (mandibular division of trigeminal nerve), accessory meningeal nerve
Foramen rotundum	V_2 (maxillary division of trigeminal nerve)
Foramen spinosum	Middle meningeal artery and vein, meningeal branch of V_3
Foramen lacerum (upper part only)	Internal carotid artery, sympathetic and venous plexuses, greater petrosal nerve (cross it)
Optic canal	Optic nerve, ophthalmic artery
Superior orbital fissure	Lacrimal, frontal, and nasociliary branches of V1 (ophthalmic branch of trigeminal nerve); oculomotor, abducent, and trochlear nerves; superior ophthalmic vein
Groove or hiatus for greater petrosal nerve	Greater petrosal nerve
Posterior cranial fossa	
Foramen magnum	Medulla oblongata, meninges and dural veins, spinal part of accessory nerves; upper cervical nerves; right and left vertebral arteries
Hypoglossal canal	Hypoglossal nerve
Internal acoustic meatus	Facial (CNVII), vestibulocochlear (CNVIII) nerves; labyrinthine artery
Jugular foramen	Glossopharyngeal (CNIX), vagus (CNX), accessory nerves (CNXI); sigmoid and inferior petrosal sinuses become internal jugular vein.

Fig. 8.6 The important openings in the base of the skull and the structures that pass through them.

- The supraorbital and supratrochlear veins unite to form the angular vein, which drains to the facial vein.
- The superficial temporal vein joins with the maxillary vein to form the retromandibular vein in the substance of the parotid salivary gland.
- The posterior auricular vein unites with the posterior division of the retromandibular vein to form the external jugular vein.
- Occipital veins drain into the suboccipital venous complex.

The scalp veins connect with the diploic veins in the skull bones and the intracranial venous sinuses by valveless emissary veins. Infections of the scalp are, therefore, potentially very serious as they may spread intracranially.

Sensory nerve supply to the scalp is shown in Fig. 8.8. The muscles of the scalp and external ear are supplied by the facial nerve.

Face

Between the skin of the face and the facial bones lies loose connective tissue. There is no deep fascia. Thus facial lacerations tend to gape open. The muscles (of facial expression) of the face lie in this connective tissue, and relatively large buccal fat pads round the skin of the cheeks. Like the scalp, the skin of the face is very sensitive and very vascular.

Sensory innervation of the face is from the trigeminal nerve (V). It has three divisions: the ophthalmic (V_1), the maxillary (V_2), and the

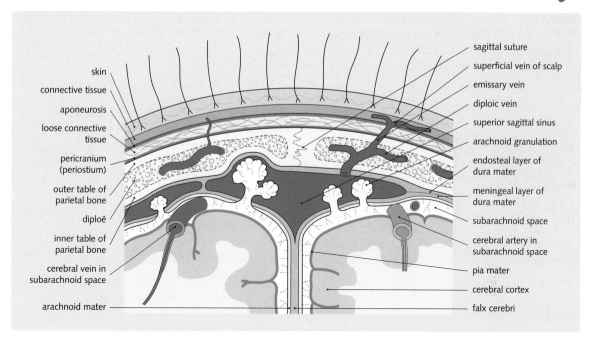

skin
connective tissue
aponeurosis
loose connective tissue
pericranium (periostium)
outer table of parietal bone
diploë
inner table of parietal bone
cerebral vein in subarachnoid space
arachnoid mater

sagittal suture
superficial vein of scalp
emissary vein
diploic vein
superior sagittal sinus
arachnoid granulation
endosteal layer of dura mater
meningeal layer of dura mater
subarachnoid space
cerebral artery in subarachnoid space
pia mater
cerebral cortex
falx cerebri

Fig. 8.7 Layers of the scalp.

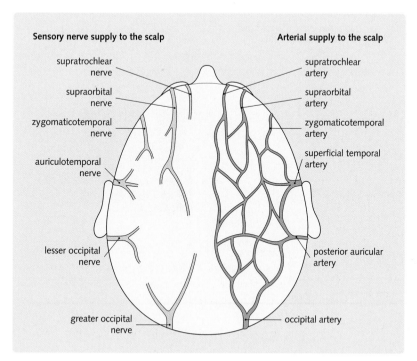

Sensory nerve supply to the scalp

Arterial supply to the scalp

supratrochlear nerve
supraorbital nerve
zygomaticotemporal nerve
auriculotemporal nerve
lesser occipital nerve
greater occipital nerve

supratrochlear artery
supraorbital artery
zygomaticotemporal artery
superficial temporal artery
posterior auricular artery
occipital artery

Fig. 8.8 Nerve and arterial supply to the scalp.

mandibular (V_3) nerves. These supply the upper, middle, and lower thirds of the face, respectively (Fig. 8.9). V_1 and V_3 are wholly sensory, while V_3 has a motor component as well, which supplies the muscles of mastication.

The order of the layers of the scalp are:
S = **S**kin
C = **C**onnective tissue
A = **A**poneurosis
L = **L**oose connective tissue
P = **P**ericranium (periostium)

Muscles of the face

Most of the muscles of facial expression are attached to the overlying skin (Fig. 8.10). They allow a wide variety of changes in facial expression to convey thought and mood. All of these muscles are supplied by the facial nerve (VII).

Vessels of the face

The face has a very rich blood supply, derived mainly from the facial, superficial temporal, and maxillary arteries, all of which are branches of the external carotid artery (Fig. 8.11).

The facial artery ascends deep to the submandibular gland, winds around the inferior border of the mandible, and enters the face. It gives off the following branches as it ascends in the face:

- The inferior labial artery.
- The superior labial artery.
- The lateral nasal artery.
- The angular artery.

The supraorbital and supratrochlear arteries are terminal branches of the ophthalmic artery—a branch of the internal carotid artery.

The facial vein is a continuation of the angular vein, which is formed by the union of the

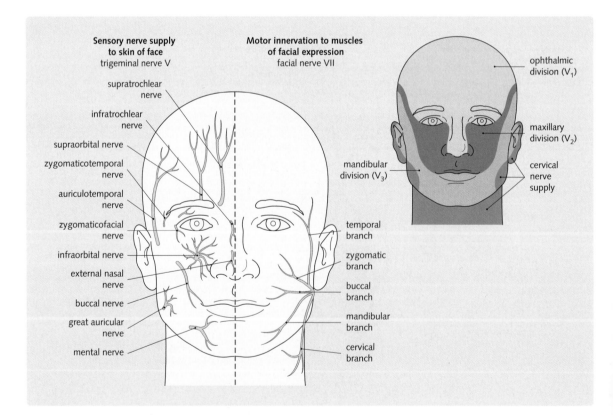

Fig. 8.9 Nerves of the face. Inset shows the distribution of the divisions of the trigeminal nerve. Note the great auricular nerve is not part of the trigeminal nerve.

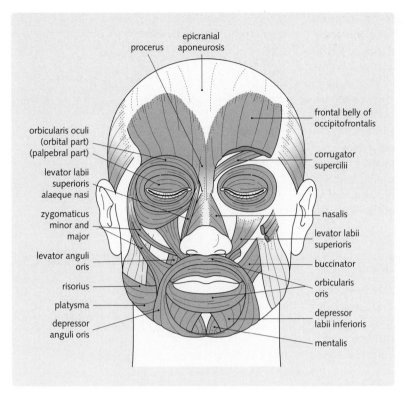

Fig. 8.10 Muscles of the face.

Labels for Fig. 8.10:
- procerus
- epicranial aponeurosis
- orbicularis oculi (orbital part) (palpebral part)
- levator labii superioris alaeque nasi
- zygomaticus minor and major
- levator anguli oris
- risorius
- platysma
- depressor anguli oris
- frontal belly of occipitofrontalis
- corrugator supercilii
- nasalis
- levator labii superioris
- buccinator
- orbicularis oris
- depressor labii inferioris
- mentalis

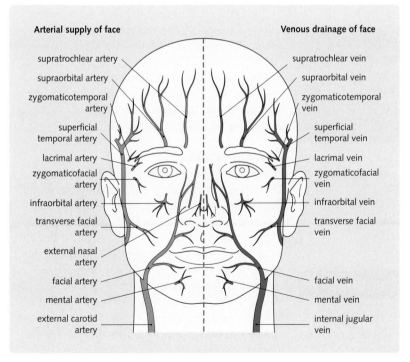

Fig. 8.11 Blood supply to the face.

Arterial supply of face
- supratrochlear artery
- supraorbital artery
- zygomaticotemporal artery
- superficial temporal artery
- lacrimal artery
- zygomaticofacial artery
- infraorbital artery
- transverse facial artery
- external nasal artery
- facial artery
- mental artery
- external carotid artery

Venous drainage of face
- supratrochlear vein
- supraorbital vein
- zygomaticotemporal vein
- superficial temporal vein
- lacrimal vein
- zygomaticofacial vein
- infraorbital vein
- transverse facial vein
- facial vein
- mental vein
- internal jugular vein

supraorbital and supratrochlear veins. It descends obliquely across the face and receives tributaries corresponding to the branches of the artery. It drains into the internal jugular vein.

The facial vein connects with the pterygoid plexus, infraophthalmic vein, and the cavernous sinus in the skull via the superior ophthalmic vein, thus providing a path for spread of infection from the face to the cavernous sinus. Even minor infections from acne on the sides of the nose and the upper lip can lead to serious complications. As a result, the triangular area from the bridge of the nose to the sides of the upper lip is known as the 'danger triangle.'

Motor nerve supply to the face

This is from the facial nerve (CN VII). The nerve exits the skull through the stylomastoid foramen to lie between the mastoid and styloid processes. It runs anteriorly to the parotid gland, within which it divides into its five groups of terminal branches that supply the muscles of facial expression (see Fig. 8.10).

Before entering the parotid gland the facial nerve gives off the posterior auricular nerve to the auricle of the ear, with motor fibers to the occipital belly of occipitofrontalis, the stylohyoid muscle, the posterior belly of the digastric muscle, and the posterior auricular muscle.

For branches of the facial nerve to the face, use the following mnemonic: **To Z**anzibar **B**y **M**otor **C**ar (**t**emporal, **z**ygomatic, **b**uccal, **m**andibular, **c**ervical).

Lymphatic drainage of the face

The lymph vessels of the face all drain into a pericervical ring of lymph nodes that then drain to the deep cervical nodes (Fig. 8.12).

The cranial cavity and meninges

The cranium protects the brain, its surrounding meninges, the proximal cranial nerves, and the vasculature of the brain. The outer surface of the

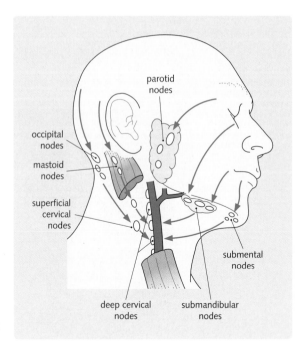

Fig. 8.12 Lymphatic drainage of the face.

cranial bones is covered by the pericranium, the inner surface by the endocranium. The two layers are continuous at the interlocking fibrous sutures of the skull.

The cranial bones consist of outer and inner tables of compact bone separated by cancellous bone containing red marrow—the diploë (see Fig. 8.7).

The base of the skull forms the floor on which the brain lies. The internal surface of the base may be divided into the anterior, middle, and posterior cranial fossae (Fig. 8.13).

Cranial fossae
Features of the anterior cranial fossa

The anterior cranial fossa is formed by the frontal and ethmoid bones and the lesser wings of the sphenoids. Behind the posterior extension of the frontal bone (frontal crest) is the foramen cecum, a passage for vessels in the fetus. Posteriorly, the axons of the olfactory nerves pass through the cribiform plate of the ethmoid bone along with the anterior ethmoid nerve. The crista galli projects from the cribiform plate.

The anterior cranial fossa contains the frontal lobes of the brain and the olfactory bulbs.

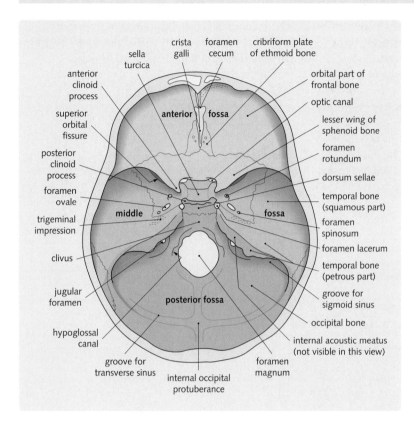

Fig. 8.13 Internal surface of the base of the skull, showing the cranial fossae.

Features of the middle cranial fossa

The middle cranial fossa is formed by the greater and lesser wings of the sphenoid bones and the squamous and petrous part of the temporal bones. The middle cranial fossa is separated from the anterior fossa by the sphenoid crests and from the posterior fossa by the superior edges of the petrous ridges of the temporal bones. The sella turcica is a saddle-like depression on the upper body of the sphenoid, surrounded by the anterior and posterior clinoid processes. A shallow depression (trigeminal impression) near the medial end of the petrous ridge houses the ganglion of CN V.

The middle cranial fossa contains the temporal lobes of the cerebral hemispheres, the floor of the forebrain, the optic chiasma, the termination of the internal carotid arteries, and the pituitary gland.

The pituitary gland lies in the pituitary fossa of the sella turcica, below the optic chiasma. In addition to endocrine problems, a tumor of the pituitary gland may compress the chiasma, creating visual problems.

Features of the posterior cranial fossa

The posterior cranial fossa is composed mainly of the occipital bone, with the petrous and mastoid portions of the temporal bone laterally and the dorsum sellae of the sphenoid bone anteriorly. From the dorsum sellae there is an incline, the clivus, leading to the foramen magnum. Posteriorly the internal occipital crest terminates at the internal occipital protuberance, separating the cerebellar fossae. Broad grooves show the location of the transverse and sigmoid sinuses. The posterior cranial fossa is roofed by the tentorium cerebelli layer of the dura mater. It contains the pons, medulla, and cerebellum.

The foramina in the cranial fossae and their main contents are outlined in Fig. 8.6.

Meninges

There are three meningeal layers surrounding the brain and spinal cord (see Fig. 8.7):
- The dura mater.
- The arachnoid mater.
- The pia mater.

Dura mater

The dura mater may be divided into two layers:

- The external periosteal layer is the endosteum lining the inner surface of the cranial bones.
- The meningeal layer (the dura mater proper) is made up of dense, strong fibrous tissue. It is continuous with the dura mater of the spinal cord at the foramen magnum. The dura sends sleeves around the cranial nerves, which fuse with the epineurium of the nerves outside the skull.

The meningeal layer of dura mater gives rise to four infoldings that form partial partitions between parts of the brain and support other parts:

- The falx cerebri.
- The tentorium cerebelli.
- The falx cerebelli.
- The diaphragma sellae.

Falx cerebri

This is a sickle-shaped fold of dura that separates the two cerebral hemispheres (Fig. 8.14). It is attached anteriorly to the internal frontal crest and

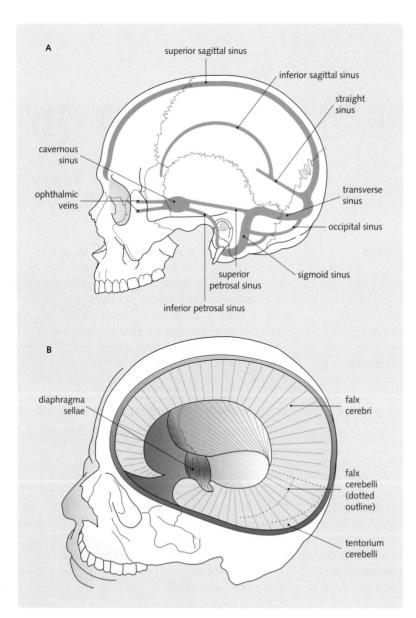

Fig. 8.14 (A) The positions of the cranial venous sinuses. (B) The falx cerebri, falx cerebelli, diaphragma sellae, and tentorium cerebelli.

the crista galli. Posteriorly, it is continuous with the tentorium cerebelli.

The superior sagittal sinus runs in its superior margin, which is attached to the calvaria along its internal midline and ends posteriorly at the confluence of sinuses (superior sagittal, straight, transverse, and occipital sinuses). The inferior sagittal sinus runs in its inferior free margin and ends in the straight sinus, which runs along the attachment of the falx to the tentorium cerebelli.

Tentorium cerebelli
This is a crescent-shaped fold of dura mater that roofs the posterior cranial fossa (see Fig. 8.14). It separates the cerebellum from the occipital lobes of the cerebral hemispheres, which it supports. The brainstem passes through an anterior gap called the tentorial notch.

The tentorium is attached to the anterior clinoid process anteriorly, the petrous ridge of the temporal bone anterolaterally, and to the occipital and parietal bones posterolaterally. Posteriorly the falx cerebri and falx cerebelli are attached to its upper and lower surfaces.

The superior petrosal and transverse venous sinuses run along its attachment to the petrous and occipital bones, respectively.

Falx cerebelli
This is a dural infolding attached to the internal occipital crest. It partially separates the two cerebellar hemispheres. Its attached posterior margin contains the occipital sinus.

Diaphragma sellae
This is a small circular fold of dura suspended between the anterior and posterior clinoid processes, which forms the roof of the pituitary fossa.

Arachnoid mater
The arachnoid mater surrounds the brain. It is applied to the dura but may be separated from the dura mater by bleeding into the subdural (potential) space, and it is separated from the pia mater by the subarachnoid space, which contains cerebrospinal fluid, arteries, and veins.

Where the arachnoid bridges major infoldings of the brain surface, the subarachnoid space expands to form subarachnoid cisterns containing cerebrospinal fluid.

Pia mater
The pia mater is a highly vascularized membrane that closely invests the brain surface. It continues as a sheath around the small vessels entering the brain. Fine, web-like arachnoid trabeculae attach the arachnoid to the pia. In some areas the pia invaginates into the ventricles, forming the choroid plexuses, which secrete cerebrospinal fluid.

Nerve supply of the meninges
Dura mater of the floors of the anterior and middle cranial fossae and of the roof of the posterior cranial fossa is supplied by neningeal branches of the trigeminal nerve. The dura of the floor of the posterior fossa is supplied by the C2 and C3 nerves, and meningeal branches of the vagal and hypoglossal nerves.

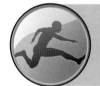

Neck pain can be referred to the head due to the upper three cervical nerves supplying the dura mater posteriorly.

Cranial venous sinuses
The cranial venous sinuses are membrane-lined spaces between the periosteal and meningial layers of the dura mater. They are valveless (see Fig. 8.14). Tributaries from cerebral veins, emissary veins, and veins from the diploë, the orbit, and the inner ear drain into these sinuses.

Superior sagittal sinus
The superior sagittal sinus runs in the convex upper border of the falx cerebri. It commences at the foramen cecum and passes backwards, grooving the calvaria of the skull. At the internal occipital protuberance, it contributes to the confluence of the sinuses. It receives numerous superior cerebral veins and communicates with lateral venous lacunae, within which are found accumulations of arachnoid granulations (see Fig. 8.7).

Inferior sagittal sinus
The inferior sagittal sinus lies in the concave free margin of the falx cerebri. At the free margin of the tentorium cerebelli it joins the great cerebral vein to form the straight sinus.

Straight sinus

The straight sinus lies along the line of attachment of the falx cerebri to the tentorium cerebelli. It ends by contributing to the confluence of sinuses.

Transverse sinuses

The transverse sinuses commence at the confluence of sinuses and run laterally in the attached margin of the tentorium cerebelli. They end by turning inferiorly as the sigmoid sinuses. They receive the superior petrosal sinuses and the cerebral, cerebellar, and diploic veins.

Sigmoid sinuses

Each sigmoid sinus follows an S-shaped path downward and medially, forming deep grooves in the temporal and occipital bones. It then turns downward through the posterior part of the jugular foramen to become continuous with the superior bulb of the internal jugular vein.

Occipital sinus

The occipital sinus lies in the attached margin of the falx cerebelli. It drains into the confluence of sinuses and communicates inferiorly with the internal vertebral venous plexus.

Cavernous sinuses

The cavernous sinuses lie on either side of the sella turcica on the body of the sphenoid. Each consists of a very thin-walled venous plexus that extends from the superior orbital fissure anteriorly to the apex of the petrous temporal bone posteriorly.

They receive:
- The superior and inferior ophthalmic veins.
- The superior and middle cerebral veins.
- The sphenoparietal sinus.
- The central vein of the retina.

They drain posteriorly into the superior and inferior petrosal sinuses and inferiorly into the pterygoid venous plexus. The two sinuses communicate via anterior and posterior intercavernous sinuses.

Relations of the cavernous sinuses

The internal carotid artery with its surrounding sympathetic nerve plexus and the abducens nerve run through the sinus (Fig. 8.15). The oculomotor (CN III) and trochlear (CN IV) nerves and the ophthalmic (CN V_1) and maxillary (CN V_2) divisions of the trigeminal nerves are embedded in the lateral wall of the sinus, between the endothelium and the dura.

Superior and inferior petrosal sinuses

The superior and inferior petrosal sinuses lie at the superior crest and inferior margin of the petrous part of the temporal bone, respectively.

Each superior sinus drains the cavernous sinus into the transverse sinus. Each inferior sinus drains the cavernous sinus into the origin of the internal jugular vein.

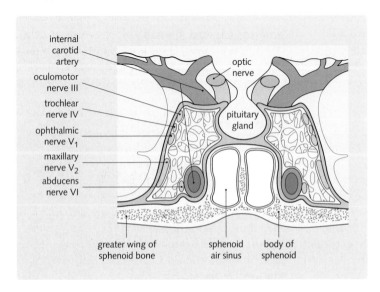

Fig. 8.15 A coronal section of the cavernous sinus showing its relations.

Parts of the brain

Although the anatomy of the brain is the purview of the fields of neuroanatomy, some knowledge is essential to understanding the organization of the dural folds, the relationship of the cavities of the skull to the different parts of the brain, the circulation of cerebrospinal fluid, and the origin of the cranial nerves. The prinicpal parts of the brain are:

- The forebrain, which is comprised of the cerebrum or cerebral hemispheres, containing the right and left ventricles, and the diencephalon, containing the third ventricle.
- The midbrain, containing the cerebral aqueduct.
- The hindbrain, which is comprised of the pons, medulla oblongata, and the cerebellum, and which contains the fourth ventricle.

The bulk of the brain is composed of the cerebral hemispheres. They are separated by the longitudinal cerebral fissure, into which projects the falx cerebri. They occupy the anterior and middle cranial fossae and extend posteriorly over the cerebellum, but are separated from it by the tentorium cerebelli. The surface layer of each hemisphere, or cortex, is thrown into folds, or gyri, separated by grooves, or sulci. The two hemispheres are connected by the corpus callosum (Fig. 8.16).

The diencephalon is composed of a dorsal thalamus and a ventral hypothalamus. The hypothalamus forms the floor and part of the lateral walls of the third ventricle, and the optic chiasm and infundibulum (which is continuous with the neural hypophysis—the posterior lobe of the pituitary) are found in the floor.

The midbrain is the narrow part of the brain that passes through the tentorial notch and connects the forebrain and the hindbrain. Running through it is the cerebral aqueduct that connects the third and fourth ventricles. The midbrain, pons, and medulla comprise the brainstem.

The pons is the most rostral part of the hindbrain, and it lies below the midbrain and above the medulla in the anterior part of the posterior cranial fossa. It is composed primarily of fibers connecting the two halves of the cerebellum, and the superior part of the fourth ventricle lies within it.

The medulla oblongata is the most caudal part of the brainstem and is continuous with the spinal cord. Within it is the inferior part of the fourth ventricle, which is continuous with the cerebral aqueduct above and the spinal canal below.

The cerebellum consists of paired lateral parts, the cerebellar hemispheres, and a small midline portion, the vermis, continuous with both hemispheres. It lies beneath the tentorium cerebelli in the posterior cranial fossa.

Eight of the twelve cranial nerves (see Fig. 8.18) arise from the brain.

Circulation of cerebrospinal fluid

Cerebrospinal fluid (CSF), a product of the choroids plexuses in the ventricles, fills the ventricles and arachnoid spaces in the brain and spinal cord and is essential to the normal function of the brain. CSF leaves the lateral ventricles in the cerebral hemispheres through the interventricular foramina and enters the third ventricle. It then passes through the cerebral aqueduct into the fourth ventricle and enters the subarachnoid space via the ventricle's median and lateral apertures.

CSF also flows into subarachnoid cisterns, areas where the pia and the arachnoid duras are widely separated and which can contain arteries, veins, and the roots of cranial nerves.

Lobes of the brain		
Lobe	Location	Extent
Frontal	Anterior cranial fossa	From frontal pole to central sulcus
Temporal	Lateral part of anterior cranial fossa	Below lateral sulcus
Occipital	Posterior cranial fossa on tentorium cerebri	From parieto-occipital sulcus to occipital pole
Parietal	Middle and posterior cranial fossa	From central sulcus to parieto-occipital sulcus

Fig. 8.16 Description of lobes of the brain.

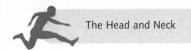

CSF is absorbed into the venous system via the arachnoid granulations, collections of finger-like projections of the arachnoid (villi) in the walls of the dural venous sinuses.

Arteries of the brain

The brain is supplied by the two internal carotid arteries and the two vertebral arteries, which lie in the subarachnoid space.

Internal carotid artery

The internal carotid artery is a terminal branch of the common carotid artery, which arises in the neck (Fig. 8.17). It enters the skull through the carotid canal and emerges from the canal above the foramen lacerum (which is sealed by a cartilaginous plate) to enter the middle cranial fossa. It crosses the superior end of the foramen lacerum and runs forward within the cavernous sinus. At the anterior end of the sinus, below the anterior clinoid process, it turns superiorly and pierces the roof. It then enters the subarachnoid space and its cerebral part turns posteriorly to join the arterial circle of Willis. Here, it divides into the anterior and middle cerebral arteries.

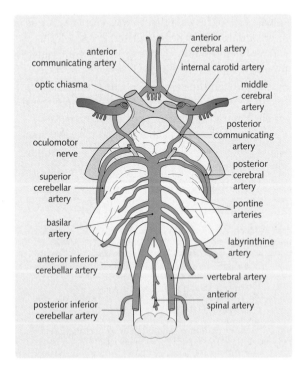

Fig. 8.17 Internal carotid and vertebral arteries on the base of the brain.

Branches of the internal carotid include:
- The ophthalmic artery.
- The posterior communicating artery.
- The choroidal artery.
- The anterior cerebral artery.
- The middle cerebral artery.

Vertebral artery

This arises from the first part of the subclavian artery. It ascends in the transverse foramina of the upper six cervical vertebrae, perforates the dura, and enters the skull through the foramen magnum. It passes upwards on the medulla oblongata (see Fig. 8.17), and it joins the vessel from the opposite side to form the basilar artery at the caudal border of the pons.

The major cranial branches of the vertebral artery include:
- The anterior and posterior spinal arteries.
- The posterior inferior cerebellar artery.
- The medullary arteries.

Basilar artery

The basilar artery ascends on the clivus to the superior border of the pons, where it divides into the posterior cerebral arteries. It also gives off branches to the pons, cerebellum, and internal ear (see Fig. 8.17).

 Plaque formation (atherosclerosis) in a vertebral artery can result in impaired blood flow to the brain (vertebrobasilar insuffiency). Impairing blood flow can be caused by hyperextension of the neck, which blocks the atherosclerotic artery and causes fainting (syncope).

Cerebral arterial circle

The cerebral arterial circle (of Willis) is a roughly circular anastomosis between branches of the internal carotid arteries and the vertebral arteries (see Fig. 8.17). It lies at the base of the brain. It allows blood entering either the carotid or vertebral artery to be shunted to any part of both cerebral hemispheres. Parts of the circle may vary in size.

Ischemic strokes or cerebrovascular accidents are common neurological disorders in adults in the USA. They are generally caused by an embolism in a major cerebral artery. If the anastomoses between the cerebral vessels of the arterial circle are not sufficient to supply the tissue directly affected by the blockage, death of that part of the brain may result.

Cranial nerves

The cranial nerves (CN) are summarized in Fig. 8.18.

Summary of cranial nerves	
Nerve	**Distribution and functions**
Olfactory (I)	Smell from nasal mucosa of root and superior sides of each nasal cavity
Optic (II)	Vision from retina
Oculomotor (III)	Motor to all extrinsic eye muscles except superior oblique and lateral rectus; parasympathetic innervation to sphincter papillae and ciliary muscle (constricts pupil and accommodates lens of eye) carries sympathetic nerve fibers to smooth muscle part of levator palpebrae superioris
Trochlear (IV)	Motor to superior oblique
Trigeminal (V) Ophthalmic division (V$_1$) Maxillary division (V$_2$) Mandibular division (V$_3$)	 Sensation from skin of upper third of face, including cornea, scalp, eyelids, and paranasal sinuses Sensation from skin of middle third of face, including upper lip, maxillary teeth, mucosa of nose, maxillary sinuses, and palate; supplies dura mater anteriorly Motor to muscles of mastication, mylohyoid, anterior belly of digastric, tensor veli palatini, and tensor tympani; sensation from skin of lower third of face, including temporomandibular joint, mucosa of mouth, and anterior two-thirds of tongue; supplies dura mater anteriorly
Abducent (VI)	Motor to lateral rectus
Facial (VII)	Motor to muscles of facial expression and scalp, stapedius, stylohyoid, and posterior belly of digastric; taste from anterior two-thirds of tongue, floor of mouth, and palate; sensation from skin of external acoustic meatus; parasympathetic innervation to submandibular and sublingual salivary glands, lacrimal gland, and glands of nose and palate
Vestibulocochlear (VIII)	Vestibular sensation from semicircular ducts, utriole, and saccule; hearing from spiral organ
Glossopharyngeal (IX)	Motor to stylopharyngeus, parasympathetic innervation to protid gland; visceral sensation from parotid gland, carotid body and sinus, pharynx, and middle ear; taste and general sensation from posterior third of tongue
Vagus (X)	Motor to constrictor muscles of pharynx, intrinsic muscles of pharynx, and muscles of palate (except tensor veli palatini) and superior two-thirds of esophagus; parasympathetic innervation to smooth muscle of trachea, bronchi, digestive tract, and cardiac muscle of heart; visceral sensation from pharynx, larynx, trachea, bronchi, heart, esophagus, stomach, and intestine to left colic flexure; taste from epiglottis and palate; sensation from auricle, external acoustic meatus, and dura mater of posterior cranial fossa
Accessory (XI) Cranial root Spinal root	 Motor to striated muscle of soft palate, pharynx, and larynx via fibers that join X in jugular foramen Motor to sternocleidomastoid and trapezius
Hypoglossal (XII)	Sensory to dura mater, posteriorly; motor to intrinsic and extrinsic muscles of tongue (except palatoglossus)

Fig. 8.18 Summary of cranial nerves.

The orbit

The eyeball and its associated muscles, nerves, and vessels are protected by the bony orbital cavity. The mobile eyelids control exposure of the eyes anteriorly.

Eyelids

The eyelids are two mobile folds of skin lying in front of the eyeball, separated from each other by the palpebral fissure and from the eyeball by the conjunctival sac (Fig. 8.19). The superficial surface of the lids is covered by the skin; the deep surface is covered by mucosa—the palpebral conjunctiva. The junctions of the superior and inferior eyelids create the angles of the eye.

The secretions of the tarsal and ciliary glands in the eyelid lubricate the eyelids and keep them from sticking together.

The triangular space at the medial angle of the eye where tears collect is called the lacrimal lake. The lacrimal glands lie in the fossae in the superolateral part of each orbit. Tears are secreted via 8–12 lacrimal ducts into the superior recess (fornix) of the conjunctival sac and are continually spread over the conjunctiva and cornea by blinking, preventing damage to the eye. The tears then collect in the lacrimal lake and drain via the lacrimal punctum, or opening, on the lacrimal papilla, which is located in the area of the lake. From there, tears enter the lacrimal canaliculi, or small canals, that drain into the lacrimal sac. This sac is the upper blind end of the nasolacrimal duct, which drains the tears into the inferior meatus of the nose.

The nerve supply to the lacrimal gland is both parasympathetic and sympathetic. Parasympathetic, or secretomotor, fibers originate in the lacrimal nucleus. Parasympathetic fibers travel in the facial nerve, greater petrosal nerve, then the nerve of the pterygoid canal to synapse in the pterygopalatine ganglion. Vasoconstrictive postganglionic sympathetic fibers from the superior cervical ganglion, via the internal carotid plexus and the deep petrosal nerve, join the nerve of the pterygoid canal to reach the pterygopalatine fossa. The postganglionic parasympathetic and sympathetic fibers now join the zygomaticotemporal nerve (a V_2 branch), then travel via the lacrimal nerve (a V_1 branch) before supplying the lacrimal gland.

The upper and lower eyelids are stengthened by plates of dense connective tissue called the tarsal plates (Fig. 8.20). The medial and lateral palpebral ligaments attach the tarsi to the medial and lateral margins of the orbit, respectively. The orbicularis oculi muscle originates and inserts onto the medial palpebral ligament. The levator palpebrae superioris muscle is attached to the superior tarsal plate. A weak connectvie tissue (orbital) septum runs from the margins of the orbit to the tarsi.

The palpebral conjunctiva is the mucous membrane lining the eyelid. It is reflected at the superior and inferior fornices (recesses), where it is continuous with the bulbar conjunctiva on the

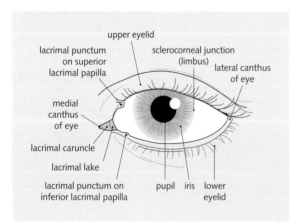

Fig. 8.19 Eyelids, palpebral fissure, and eyeball.

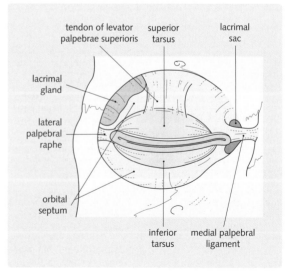

Fig. 8.20 Orbital septum, tarsi, and palpebral ligaments.

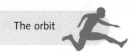

anterior surface of the eyeball. The palpebral and bulbar conjunctiva form the conjunctival sac when the eyes are closed (Fig. 8.21).

Orbital cavity

Fig. 8.22 illustrates the bony components of the orbital cavity, which resembles a quadrangular pyramid.

The orbital cavity boundaries are as follows:
• Superiorly (roof)—frontal bone (orbital part), lesser wing of sphenoid bone. It contains the fossa for the lacrimal gland.
• Medial wall—mainly the ethmoid bone, with contributions from the lacrima and frontal bones and the body of sphenoid bone. It is indented by the lacrimal groove and the fossa of the lacrimal sac.
• Inferiorly (floor)—maxillary bone, zygomatic bone, palatine bone. It contains the inferior orbital fissure.
• Lateral wall—zygomatic bone (frontal process), greater wing of sphenoid bone.
• Apex of the orbit—lesser wing of the sphenoid bone. It contains the optic canal and the superior orbital fissure.

Fig. 8.23 shows the orbital openings and their contents.

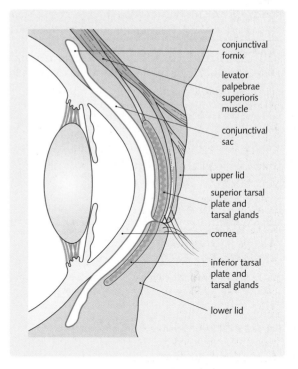

Fig. 8.21 Conjunctival sac, upper and lower lids, and cornea.

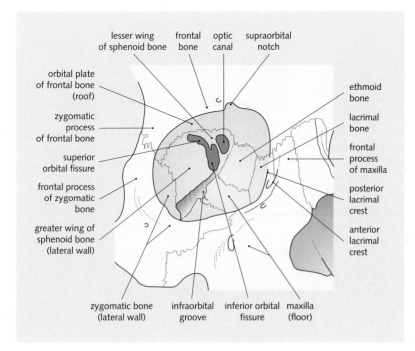

Fig. 8.22 Bones of the orbit.

Orbital openings and their contents

Opening	Bones	Contents
Supraorbital notch (foramen)	Orbital palate of the frontal bone	Supraorbital nerve and vessels
Infraorbital groove and canal	Orbital palate of the maxilla	Infraorbital nerve and vessels
Inferior orbital fissure	Maxilla and greater wing of the sphenoid bone	Communicates with pterygopalatine fossa and transmits the infraorbital and zygomatic nerves, the inferior ophthalmic vein, and sympathetic nerves
Superior orbital fissure	Greater and lesser wing of the sphenoid bone	Lacrimal, frontal, trochlear, oculomotor, abducens, and nasociliary nerves, and superior ophthalmic vein
Optic canal	Lesser wing of the spheniod bone	Optic nerve and ophthalmic artery
Zygomaticotemporal and zygomaticofacial foramina	Zygomatic bone	Zygomaticotemporal and zygomaeticofacial nerves from the zygomatic nerve
Anterior and posterior ethmoid foramina	Ethmoid bone and orbital plate of frontal bone	Anterior and posterior ethmoidal nerves and vessels

Fig. 8.23 Orbital openings and their contents.

The eyeball

The eyball consists of three layers:

- A fibrous outer coat consisting of the sclera and cornea.
- A middle vascular layer of the choroids, ciliary body, and iris.
- An inner coat consisting of both visual and nonvisual parts of the retina.

The sclera is the white part of the eye. The anterior one-sixth of it is the cornea, which is transparent.

The choroid forms most of the vascular layer, and consists of a pigmented vascular bed that lies adjacent to the avascular, visual area of the retina. The choroid provides oxygen and nutrients to the retina. The ciliary body connects the choroid with the circumference of the iris and attaches to the lens via the smooth ciliary muscles that control the thickness of the lens, e.g., the focus. The ciliary processes, folds on the internal surface of the ciliary body, produce aqueous humor. The iris lies on the anterior surface of the lens, and contains two involuntary muscles controlled by autonomic innervation: the parasympathetically stimulated sphincter pupillae and the sympathetically stimulated dilator pupillae. These muscles close and open the pupil, respectively. The pupil is the central aperture in the iris that transmits light.

The optic or visual part of the retina consists of two layers: the neural layer, which is light sensitive, and the pigmented layer, which reinforces the light-absorbing properties of the choroid. The nonvisual part of the retina is a continuation of the pigmented layer over the ciliary body and the posterior surface of the iris.

Aqueous humor, produced by the ciliary processes of the ciliary body, is a clear, watery solution that provides nutrients to the avascular cornea and lens. It fills the anterior and posterior chambers of the eye. The anterior chamber is the space between the cornea anteriorly and the lens and ciliary body posteriorly. Vitreous humor is found within the meshwork of the vitreous body, a jelly-like substance in the large chamber of the eyeball, posterior to the lens. It transmits light and holds the retina in place.

Muscles of the orbit

The muscles of the orbit are outlined in Fig. 8.24 and illustrated in Fig. 8.25. The four rectus muscles arise from the common tendinous ring surrounding the optic canal and part of the superior orbital fissure.

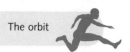

| Muscles of the eyeballs and eyelids ||||
Name of muscle (nerve supply)	Origin	Insertion	Action
Extrinsic muscles of eyeball (striated skeletal muscle)			
Superior rectus (CNIII)	Common tendinous ring on posterior wall of orbital cavity	Superior surface of eyeball just posterior to corneoscleral junction	Elevates, adducts, and rotates eyeball upward and medially
Inferior rectus (CNIII)	Common tendinous ring on posterior wall of orbital cavity	Inferior surface of eyeball just posterior to corneoscleral junction	Depresses, adducts, and rotates eyeball laterally and medially
Medial rectus (CNIII)	Common tendinous ring on posterior wall of orbital cavity	Medial surface of eyeball just posterior to corneoscleral junction	Adducts eyeball so that the eye looks medially
Lateral rectus (CNVI)	Common tendinous ring on posterior wall of orbital cavity	Lateral surface of eyeball just posterior to corneoscleral junction	Adducts eyeball so that the eye looks laterally
Superior oblique (CNIV)	Body of sphenoid bone	Passes through a fibrous ring or trochlea and is attached to superior surface of eyeball deep to superior rectus, behind the equator	Adducts, depresses, and rotates eyeball so that the the eye looks downward and laterally
Inferior oblique (CNIII)	Anterior floor of oral cavity	Lateral surface of eyeball deep to lateral rectus	Adducts, elevates, and rotates eyeball so that the eye looks upward and laterally
Intrinsic muscles of eyeball (smooth muscles)			
Sphincter pupillae of iris (parasympathetic via CNIII)	Ring of smooth muscle passing circumferentially around inner edge of iris		Constricts pupil
Dilator pupillae of iris (sympathetic)	Radially oriented smooth muscle fibers from the outer edge of the iris	Sphincter pupillae	Dilates pupil
Ciliary muscle (parasympthetic via CNIII)	Smooth muscle within the ciliary body	Ciliary body	Controls shape of lens; in accommodation, makes more convex to increase depth of focus
Muscles of eyelids			
Orbicularis oculi (CNVII)	Medial palpebral ligament, lacrimal bone, medial margin of the orbit	Skin around orbit, tarsal plates	Closes eyelids
Levator palpebrae superioris (striated muscle: CNIII; smooth muscle, sympathetic)	Lesser ring of sphenoid bone, superior and anterior to optic canal	Superior tarsal plate and adjacent skin	Raises upper lid

Fig. 8.24 Muscles of the eyeballs and eyelids.

To recall the superior oblique muscle's action remember: 'It's the poor man's muscles, pulling the eye down and out.'

and, posteriorly, it drains to the cavernous sinus. The inferior ophthalmic vein enters the orbit via the inferior orbital tissue and communicates with the cavernous sinus and the pterygoid venous plexus.

Vessels of the orbit

Fig. 8.26 shows the arterial supply to the orbit.

The venous drainage is via the superior and inferior ophthalmic veins. The superior ophthalmic vein communicates anteriorly with the facial vein

Nerves of the orbit
Optic nerve (II)

The optic nerve is surrounded by the three meningeal layers and the subarachnoid space, extending from the brain to the eyeball. The fibers

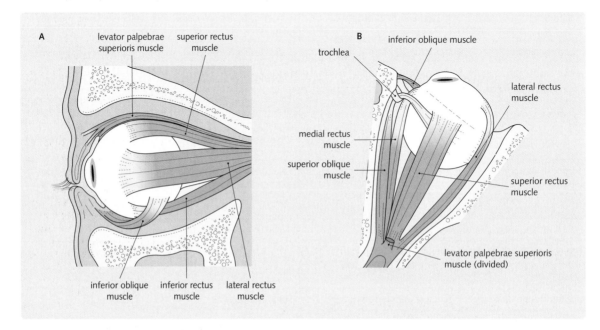

Fig. 8.25 Muscles of the orbit seen laterally (A) and from above (B).

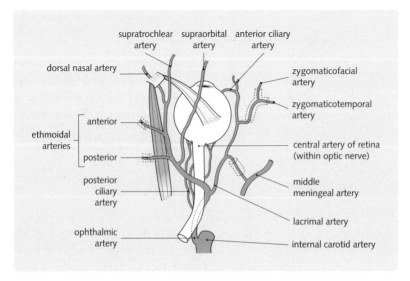

Fig. 8.26 Arterial supply to the orbit. Branches of the ophthalmic artery.

of the optic nerve are unmylenated axons from the retinal ganglion cells. These axons pierce the sclera of the eyeball and become myelinated in the region of the optic disc, then pass posteromedially in the orbit within the ring of the ocular muscles to exit via the optic canal. Fibers from the nasal half of each retina cross to the opposite side at the optic chiasm and then pass via the optic tracts to the thalamus.

Lacrimal nerve

The lacrimal nerve is a branch of the ophthalmic division of the trigeminal nerve (V_1). It passes along the upper part of the lateral rectus muscle to supply the skin of the upper lateral eyeball. It is joined by a branch of the zygomaticotemporal nerve (carrying parasympathetic fibers) to innervate the lacrimal gland.

Frontal nerve

The frontal nerve is also a branch of V_1. It passes forward on the superior surface of levator palpebrae superioris. Just before it reaches the orbital margin, it divides into the supraorbital and supratrochlear nerves, which supply the skin of the forehead and scalp, and the mucous membrane of the frontal sinus.

Nasociliary nerve

A branch of V_1, the nasociliary nerve enters the orbit between the superior and inferior divisions of the oculomotor nerve from the cavernous sinus. It crosses above the optic nerve with the ophthalmic artery within the common tendinous ring to reach the medial wall of the orbit, giving off two delicate ciliary nerves that enter the eyeball. These carry afferent fibers from the eyeball and sympathetic fibers from the carotid plexus. It runs forward on the upper margin of medial rectus, and it ends by dividing into the anterior, and occasionally a posterior, ethmoidal nerves, and the infratrochlear nerve (Fig. 8.27).

Trochlear nerve (IV)

The trochlear nerve emerges from the dorsum of the midbrain and wraps around the brainstem to reach the cavernous sinus. It leaves the lateral wall of the cavernous sinus to enter the orbit via the superior orbital fissure. It runs forward and medially across the origin of levator palpebrae superioris to the superior oblique muscle, which it supplies.

Branches of the nasociliary nerve	
Branch	Action
Communicating branch	Communicates with the ciliary ganglion—general sensory (afferent) fibers from the eyeballs pass to the ciliary ganglion via the short ciliary nerves and then to the nasociliary nerve via the communicating branch
Long ciliary nerve	2–3 branches containing postganglionic sympathetic fibers for the dilator pupillae; runs with the short ciliary nerves and pierces the sclera to reach the ciliary body and iris
Posterior ethmoidal nerve	Exits through the posterior ethmoidal foramen to supply the mucus membrane of the ethmoidal and sphenoidal air sinuses and the nasal cavity
Infratrochlear nerve	Passes below the trochlea to supply the skin over the upper eyelid and nose, conjunctiva, and lacrimal sac
Anterior ethmoidal nerve	Exits the anterior ethmoidal foramen and enters the anterior cranial fossa on the cribriform plate of the ethmoid; then enters the nasal cavity via an opening opposite the crista galli to supply the mucosa of the nose; then supplies the skin of the nose as the external nasal nerve

Fig. 8.27 Branches of the nasociliary nerve.

Oculomotor nerve (III)

The oculomotor nerve emerges from the midbrain and enters the cavernous sinus. It passes through the superior orbital fissure, where it divides into superior and inferior divisions:

- The superior division supplies the superior rectus and levator palpebrae superioris.
- The inferior division supplies the inferior rectus, medial rectus, and inferior oblique.

The nerve to inferior oblique sends a branch to the ciliary ganglion. This carries parasympathetic fibers that reach the sphincter pupillae and ciliary muscle via the short ciliary nerves.

Abducent nerve (VI)

The abducent nerve has the longest intradural course of all the cranial nerves, emerging from between the pons and medulla and coursing over the petrous portion of the temporal bone to reach the cavernous sinus. It enters the orbit via the superior orbital fissure and supplies the lateral rectus muscle.

Ciliary ganglion

The ciliary ganglion is a parasympathetic ganglion situated posteriorly in the orbit, between the optic nerve and the lateral rectus muscle.

Preganglionic parasympathetic fibers from the Edinger–Westphal nucleus pass to the ganglion via the oculomotor nerve. Postganglionic parasympathetic fibers pass to the back of the eyeball via the short ciliary nerves.

Postganglionic sympathetic fibers (from the internal carotid plexus in the cavernous sinus) pass through the ganglion to enter the short ciliary nerves. General sensory fibers leave the ganglion via the nasociliary nerve. The long ciliary nerve also carries sympathetic and sensory fibers to the eyeball.

The parasympathetic nerves supply the constrictor pupillae and ciliary muscle; the sympathetic fibers supply the dilator pupillae.

Motor innervation of the orbit other than from the oculomotor nerve: LR_6SO_4 (**L**ateral **R**ectus—CN VI; **S**uperior **O**blique—CN IV).

The parotid region

Parotid gland

The parotid gland is the largest of the paired major salivary glands. It is wedged between the ramus of the mandible and the mastoid process (Fig. 8.28).

The gland is surrounded by a tough fibrous capsule derived from the investing layer of deep cervical fascia, the parotid sheath. The stylomandibular ligament is a thickened part of the capsule, running from the mandibular angle to the styloid process.

The parotid duct emerges from the anterior border of the gland. It crosses the masseter muscle superficially and, at the anterior border of this muscle, it turns medially to pierce the buccal fat pad and buccinator to open into the oral cavity opposite the second maxillary molar tooth. The parotid gland secretes a thin, watery saliva.

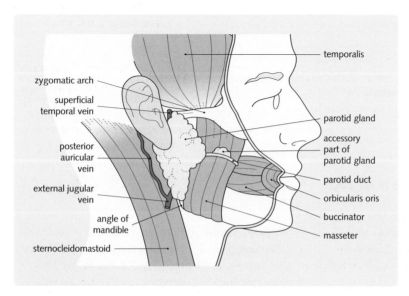

Fig. 8.28 Parotid gland and its relations. (Adapted from Clinical Anatomy For Medical Students, 4th edn., by R S Snell. Little Brown & Co.)

Structures within the parotid gland
Facial nerve (CN VII)
The facial nerve emerges from the junction of the pons and medulla. It has a motor root to the muscles of facial expression and an intermediate root, the nervus intermedius, carrying taste, parasympathetic, and somatic sensory fibers (see later discussion). It traverses the posterior cranial fossa, the internal acoustic meatus, and the facial canal in the temporal bone to emerge from the stylomastoid foramen and enter the gland, after giving off the posterior auricular nerve and muscular branches. It divides into its five terminal motor branches within the parotid gland.

 A parotid tumor compresses the facial nerve weakening the facial muscles ipsilaterally (Bell's palsy). The corner of the mouth and eye may drop.

Retromandibular vein
The retromandibular vein is formed by the union of the superficial temporal and maxillary veins and descends posterior to the ramus of the mandible through the parotid gland. It divides into anterior and posterior divisions, which leave the lower border of the gland. The anterior division joins the facial vein; the posterior division joins with the posterior auricular vein to form the external jugular vein.

External carotid artery
The external carotid artery enters the parotid gland in the neck by passing up from the carotid triangle. At the neck of the mandible it divides into its two terminal branches—the maxillary and superficial temporal arteries.

Blood supply, lymphatic drainage, and innervation of the parotid gland
Blood supply is from the external carotid artery and its terminal branches.

Parasympathetic secretomotor fibers from the inferior salivary nucleus of the glossopharyngeal nerve (IX) pass to the otic ganglion via the tympanic branch of the IX nerve and the lesser petrosal nerve. Postganglionic fibers pass to the parotid via the auriculotemporal nerve. Postganglionic sympathetic fibers come from the cervical sympathetic ganglia via the external carotid plexus. The great auricular nerve supplies sensory fibers to the parotid sheath. The great auricular and auriculotemporal nerves supply sensory fibers to the gland itself.

Parotid nodes drain the gland, forehead, external ear, and temporal region to the deep cervical nodes.

The temporal and infratemporal fossae

Temporal fossa
The temporal fossa lies on the lateral aspect of the skull. It is bounded by the superior temporal line of the temporal bone superiorly, by the frontal and zygomatic bones anteriorly, by the zygomatic arch laterally, and inferiorly by the infratemporal crest.

Contents of the temporal fossa are:
- The temporalis muscle and temporal fascia.
- The deep temporal nerves and vessels.
- The auriculotemporal nerve.
- The superficial temporal artery.

Temporal fascia
The temporal fascia covers the temporalis muscle above the zygomatic arch and roofs the temporal fossa. It is attached inferiorly to the zygomatic arch and superiorly to the superior temporal line.

Deep temporal nerves
Two or three nerves on each side arise from the mandibular nerve and emerge from the upper border of lateral pterygoid to enter and supply the temporalis muscle.

Deep temporal arteries
The deep temporal arteries are branches of the maxillary artery. They accompany the deep temporal nerves.

Auriculotemporal nerve
The auriculotemporal nerve is a branch of the posterior division of the mandibular nerve. It emerges from the upper border of the parotid

191

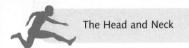

gland and crosses the root of the zygomatic arch behind the superficial temporal artery. It supplies the skin of the auricle, the external auditory meatus, and the scalp over the temporal region.

Superficial temporal artery

The superficial temporal artery emerges from behind the temporomandibular joint, crosses the zygomatic arch, and ascends to the scalp.

Infratemporal fossa

The infratemporal fossa lies deep to the zygomatic arch and the ramus of the mandible and posterior to the maxilla (Fig. 8.29). It communicates with the temporal region deep to the zygomatic arch.

The infratemporal fossa contains (Fig. 8.30):
• The medial and lateral pterygoid muscles.
• Branches of the mandibular nerve (inferior alveolar, lingual, and buccal).
• The otic ganglion.
• The chorda tympani.
• The maxillary artery.

• The pterygoid venous plexus.
• The inferior part of the temporal muscle.

Muscles of mastication

There are four large and powerful muscles of mastication (Fig. 8.31).

Boundaries of the infratemporal fossa	
Boundary	**Components**
Anterior	Posterior surface of the maxilla
Posterior	Mastoid and styloid process of temporal bone
Superior	Infratemporal surface of the greater wing of the sphenoid bone
Medial	Lateral pterygoid plate
Lateral	Ramus of the mandible

Fig. 8.29 Boundaries of the infratemporal fossa.

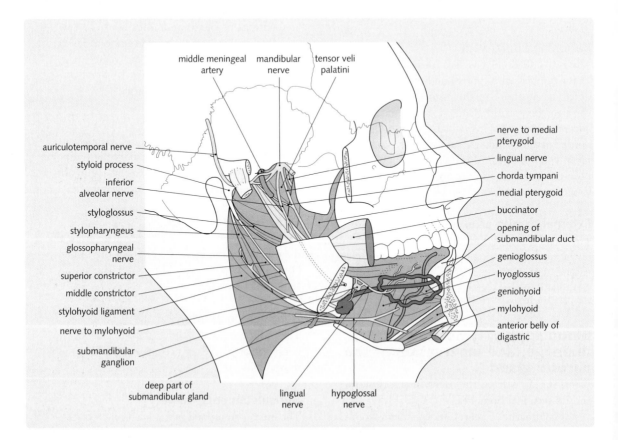

Fig. 8.30 Infratemporal fossa and its relations.

Mandible

Important features of the mandible are shown in Fig. 8.32. The two halves of the mandible unite at the midline symphysis menti.

Temporomandibular joint (TMJ)

The temporomandibular joint is the articulation between the condylar head of the mandible and the mandibular fossa of the temporal bone (Figs 8.33 and 8.34).

It is a modified hinge type of synovial joint. The joint space is divided into upper and lower compartments by an articular disc attached to the lateral pterygoid muscle anteriorly, and to the capsule of the joint.

The capsule surrounding the joint is loose, and it is attached to the margins of the mandibular fossa and the neck of the mandible. It is strengthened by the intrinsic lateral temporomandibular ligament. The stylomandibular ligament, a lateral thickening of the capsule, and the sphenomandibular ligament, which runs from the spine of the sphenoid to the lingual of the mandible, are also functionally associated with the joint.

Movements involving the TMJ include:
- Depression of the mandible (opening mouth)—gravity and suprahyoid and infrohyoid muscles, lateral pterygoid (pulls mandible forward).
- Elevation of the the mandible (closing mouth)—temporalis, masseter, medial pterygoid.
- Protrusion of the chin—lateral and medial pterygoids, masseter.
- Retraction of the chin—temporalis, masseter.
- Lateral movement (side-to-side grinding and chewing)—retractors and protruders on alternate sides.

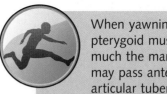

When yawning, if the lateral pterygoid muscle contracts too much the mandibular head may pass anteriorly over the articular tubercle and dislocate the temporomandibular joint. An affected individual is unable to close the mouth.

Muscles of mastication			
Muscle (nerve supply)	Origin	Insertion	Action
Temporalis (CNV₃)	Temporal fossa floor, deep surface of temporal fascia	Coronoid process and anterior border of ramus of mandible	Elevates mandible and closes jaw; posterior fibers retract a protruded mandible
Masseter (CNV₃)	Inferior border and medial surface of zygomatic arch	Lateral surface of ramus of mandible and coroniod process	Elevates and protrudes mandible, closes jaw
Lateral pterygoid (CNV) Superior head Inferior head	Infratemporal surface of sphenoid bone Lateral surface of lateral pterygoid plate	Neck of the mandible Anterior disc and capsule of TMJ	Acting together, they depress chin and protrude the mandible; acting alone and alternately, they produce side-to-side movement of the jaw
Medial pterygoid (CNV) Superficial head Deep head	Tuberosity of the maxilla Medial surface of lateral pterytoid plate, pyramidal process of palatine bone	Ramus and angle of the mandible Medial surface of ramus and angle of the mandible	Acting together, they elevate the mandible; acting alone, they protrude side of jaw; acting alternately, they produce a grinding movement

Fig. 8.31 Muscles of mastication.

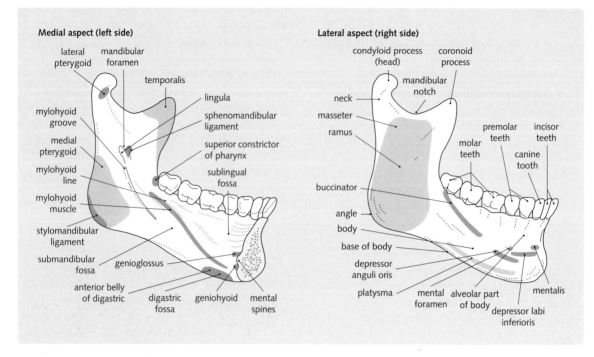

Fig. 8.32 Features of the mandible.

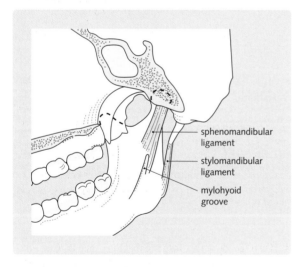

Fig. 8.33 Temporomandibular ligaments.

Fig. 8.34 Temporomandibular joint.

Mandibular nerve

Fibers from the motor and sensory roots of the trigeminal nerve form V_3, which exits the skull through the foramen ovale to enter the infratemporal fossa, where it divides into motor and sensory branches. Below the foramen ovale, the nerve is separated from the pharynx and its branches are external to the tensor veli palatine and the medial pterygoid but deep to the superior head of the lateral pterygoid muscle. After giving off a meningeal branch and the nerve to the medial pterygoid, it divides into small anterior and large anterior divisions (Fig. 8.35).

Branches of the mandibular nerve	
Branch	Area supplied
Main trunk	
Meningeal branch	Re-enters cranial cavity via foramen spinosum
Nerve to medial pterygoid	Medial pterygoid and a tiny branch that passes by otic ganglion to supply tensor tympani and tensor veli palatini
Anterior division (motor except the buccal nerve)	
Deep temporal nerves	Temporalis muscle (see temporal region)
Masseteric nerve	Passes through mandibular notch to supply masseter muscle
Nerve to lateral ptyergoid	Enters deep surface of lateral pterygoid and supplies it
Buccal nerve	Passes anteriorly between heads of lateral pterygoid to appear at anterior border of masseter; is sensory to skin of cheek and underlying buccal mucosa and gingiva
Posterior division (mainly sensory)	
Lingual nerve	Follows the inferior alveolar nerve over superior surface of medial pterygoid to run between the mandible and the spheromandibular ligament just beneath mucosa lining inner aspect of mandible adjacent to third molar tooth (its subsequent course is described later); deep to lateral pterygoid, the nerve receives the chorda tympani
Inferior alveolar nerve	Runs parallel with lingual nerve over medial pterygoid, passing between the mandible and the sphenomandibular ligament; enters mandibular foramen and supplies teeth of lower jaw; at mental foramen, a branch of the nerve, the mental nerve, exits mandible to supply lower lip and chin region; mylohyoid nerve arises from inferior alveolar nerve just above mandibular foramen to supply mylohyoid and anterior belly of digastric
Auriculotemporal nerve	Arises by two roots that encircle the middle meningeal artery; after coming together, it ascends deep to the mandible and TMJ (see temporal region for its branches)

Fig. 8.35 Branches of the mandibular nerve and the areas they supply.

Remember that the mandibular nerve is the only division of the trigeminal with voluntary motor fibers—to the muscles of mastication, the mylohyoid, the anterior belly of the digastric, the tensor veli palatini, and tensor tympani muscles.

Otic ganglion

This is a parasympathetic ganglion lying below the foramen ovale.

Preganglionic secretomotor fibers from the tympanic nerve and from the glossopharyngeal nerve (IX) join the tympanic plexus and continue as the lesser petrosal nerve to enter the otic ganglion. Here the fibers synapse and

postganglionic fibers pass via the auriculotemporal nerve to enter the parotid gland.

Sympathetic fibers from the plexus on the middle meningeal artery also pass through the ganglion, but without synapsing, to the parotid gland and its vessels.

Chorda tympani

The chorda tympani is a branch of the facial nerve in the temporal bone. It enters the infratemporal fossa via the petrotympanic fissure and joins the lingual nerve.

It transmits preganglionic parasympathetic secretomotor fibers and taste fibers from the anterior two-thirds of the tongue. Preganglionic parasympathetic fibers synapse in the submandibular ganglion and postganglionic fibers innervate the submandibular and sublingual glands. Cell bodies of the taste fibers are in the

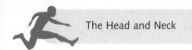

geniculate ganglion of the facial nerve and end by synapsing with cells of the nucleus solitarius in the pons.

Maxillary artery

The maxillary artery is the large terminal branch of the external carotid artery in the parotid gland. It runs forward deep to the neck of the mandible, giving off the middle meningeal and inferior alveolar arteries before entering the infratemporal fossa at the lower border of lateral pterygoid. There it gives off the masseteric artery. It then passes between the heads of lateral pterygoid, giving off the deep temporal and buccal arteries. It enters the pterygopalatine fossa through the pterygomaxillary fissure to become the superior alveolar arteries.

Fig. 8.36 shows the branches of the maxillary artery.

Pterygoid venous plexus

The pterygoid venous plexus lies around the muscles of mastication in the infratemporal fossa. It drains veins from the orbit, oral cavity, and nasal cavity. It communicates with the cavernous sinus and with the facial vein.

The pterygoid venous plexus is devoid of valves, as are all veins of the head and neck.

The ear and vestibular apparatus

The ear is the organ of hearing and balance. It may be divided into the external ear, the middle ear, and the internal ear.

Branches of the maxillary artery		
Branch	Site of origin	Area supplied
Deep auricular artery	Behind neck of mandible	TMJ, external auditory meatus, and outer surface of eardrum
Anterior tympanic artery	Behind neck of mandible	Inner surface of eardrum via petrotympanic fissure
Middle meningeal artery	Infratemporal fossa	Enters cranial cavity via foramen spinosum to supply meninges
Inferior alveolar artery	Infratemporal fossa	Follows inferior alveolar nerve into mandibulare canal and supplies lower jaw and teeth and surrounding mucosa
Deep temporal arteries	Infratemporal fossa	Muscles of mastication
Masseteric artery		
Pterygoid branches		
Posterior superior alveolar atery	Pterygopalatine fossa	Enters posterior aspect of maxilla to supply posterior molar and premolar teeth of maxilla
Infraorbital artery	From the infraorbital pterygopalantine fossa	Accompanies infraorbital nerve through infraorbital foramen onto face; reaches foramen by passing forward in infraorbital canal in orbital floor
Anterior superior alveolar artery	Infraorbital canal	Incisor and canine teeth
Descending palatine Sphenopalatine Pharyngeal branches	Pterygopalatine fossa	Described with the nasal cavity

Fig. 8.36 Branches of the maxillary artery.

External ear
Auricle
The auricle is elastic cartilage covered with skin. It collects sound, which is conducted to the tympanic membrane via the external auditory meatus.

External auditory (acoustic) meatus
The external auditory meatus extends from the auricle to the tympanic membrane (Fig. 8.37). The lateral third is cartilaginous and the medial two-thirds are bony, and the entire passage is lined by a layer of thin skin. Ceruminous and sebaceous glands produce cerumen (wax).

Tympanic membrane
The tympanic membrane is a thin membrane lying between the external ear and the tympanic cavity of the middle ear (see Fig. 8.37). It is covered by skin externally and by mucous membrane internally. The membrane shows a concavity towards the meatus, with a central, cone-like depression—the umbo. Extending superiorly is the handle and lateral process of the malleus, one of the middle ear ossicles. Superior to the lateral process, the tympanic membrane is thin and is called the pars flaccida. The rest of the membrane has radial and circular fibers and is called the pars tensa.

The membrane moves in response to air vibration. Movements are transmitted by the ossicles through the middle ear t... ear.

The auriculotemporal nerve and ... branch of the vagus supply the exter... the tympanic membrane. The glossop... nerve supplies the internal surface.

Middle ear
The middle ear lies in the petrous temporal bone. It consists of the tympanic cavity and the epitympanic recess, a space lying superior to the tympanic cavity.

It is connected to the nasopharynx via the auditory tube and to the mastoid air cells via the mastoid antrum. The mucosa lining the tympanic cavity is continuous with that of the auditory tube, mastoid cells, and the mastoid antrum.

The middle ear contains:
- The ossicles (malleus, incus, and stapes).
- Stapedius and tensor tympani muscles.
- The chorda tympani, a branch of CN VII.
- The tympanic plexus of nerves.

Fig. 8.38 describes the walls of the middle ear.

Mastoid antrum
An aditus or entrance to the antrum connects the mastoid antrum to the epitympanic recess of the tympanic cavity. A thin bony roof, the tegmen tympani, separates the antrum from the

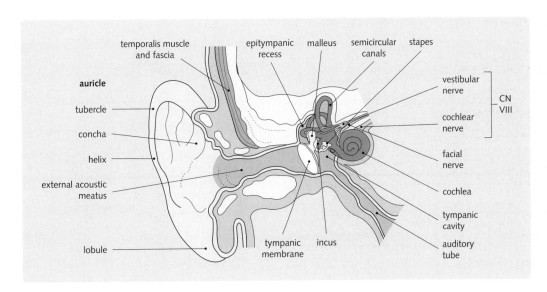

Fig. 8.37 External auditory meatus.

197

ddle cranial fossa. The floor of the antrum communicates with the mastoid air cells via several openings. The antrum and air cells are lined by mucosa. Anteroinferiorly the antrum is related to the canal for the facial nerve.

Auditory (pharyngotympanic) tube

The auditory tube connects the tympanic cavity to the nasopharynx. The posterior lateral third is bony and the remainder is cartilaginous. The mucosa is continuous with that of the tympanic cavity and nasopharynx.

It equalizes pressure in the middle ear with atmospheric pressure, allowing free movement of the tympanic membrane. Pressure changes (e.g., during flying) can be equalized by swallowing, yawning, or chewing—these movements open the auditory tubes.

Nerve supply is from the tympanic plexus formed by fibers from the glossopharyngeal and facial nerves.

The auditory tube provides a passage for infection to spread from the nasopharynx to the tympanic cavity (middle ear).

Ossicles

The ossicles are the incus, malleus, and stapes. The malleus is embedded into the tympanic membrane. The head of the malleus articulates with the body of the incus, and the long process of the incus articulates with the head of the stapes. The base of the stapes fits into the oval window on the medial wall of the tympanic cavity (Fig. 8.39).

The ossicles transmit vibration from the tympanic membrane to the oval window.

There are two muscles associated with the ossicles: the tensor tympani arises from the cartilaginous portion of the auditory tube and inserts into the handle of the malleus. By pulling on the malleus, it tenses the tympanic membrane, dampening the vibration of the tympanic membrane. The stapedius originates inside the pyramidal eminence on the posterior wall of the tympanic cavity, and inserts onto the neck of the stapes, dampening its vibrations.

They are innervated by the medial pterygoid nerve CN V_3 and VII, respectively.

Walls of the middle ear	
Wall	**Components**
Roof (tegmental wall)	Tegmen tympani (thin plate of bone); separates cavity from dura in floor of middle cranial fossa
Floor (jugular wall)	A layer of bone separates tympanic cavity from superior bulb of internal jugular vein
Lateral wall (membranous)	Tympanic membrane with epitympanic recess superiorly
Medial wall (labyrinthine)	Separates tympanic cavity from inner ear; features the promontory
Anterior wall (carotid)	Separates tympanic cavity from carotid canal; superiorly lies opening of auditory tube and canal for tensor tympani
Posterior wall	Connected by aditus to mastoid antrum and air cells

Fig. 8.38 Walls of the middle ear.

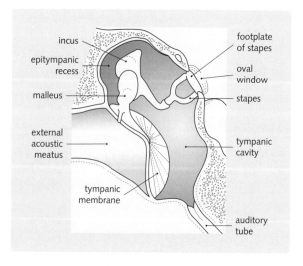

Fig. 8.39 Coronal section of the tympanic cavity showing the ossicles in situ.

Internal ear

This is buried in the petrous part of the temporal bone (Fig. 8.40). It consists of a bony labyrinth and a membranous labyrinth. The membranous labyrinth, which contains endolymph, is suspended within the bony labyrinth, which is filled with perilymph.

Bony labyrinth
Cochlea

This is a shell-shaped portion of the bony labyrinth containing the cochlear duct, and it is concerned with the reception of sound and the maintenance of equilibrium. It makes 2.5 turns about a bony core—the modiolus. The large basal turn of the cochlea produces the promontory on the medial wall of the tympanic cavity.

Vestibule

The vestibule is a small oval chamber containing the utricle and saccule, components of the balance apparatus. The oval window is on the lateral wall of the vestibule. It is continuous with the cochlea anteriorly, with the semicircular canals posteriorly, and with the posterior cranial fossa by the aqueduct of the vestibule. The aqueduct extends to the posterior surface of the petrous temporal bone to open into the internal auditory meatus. It transmits the endolymphatic ducts and tiny blood vessels.

Semicircular canals

These three (anterior, posterior, and lateral) communicate with the vestibule, and they are set at right angles to one other. At one end of each canal is a swelling—the ampulla. The semicircular ducts lie within the canals.

Membranous labyrinth

This is a communicating series of ducts and sacs in the bony labyrinth, which contain endolymph.

Cochlear labyrinth

This is a spiral blind tube, the cochlear duct (of Corti). The duct is suspended across the canal between the spiral ligament and the osseus spiral lamina, which run the length of the canal. This divides the canal into two channels, the scala vestibuli and the scala tympani, both of which are filled with perilymph and which communicate with each other at the tip of the cochlea. The receptor of auditory stimuli is the spiral organ of Corti, which is situated on the floor of the duct in the basilar membrane.

Saccule and utricle

These have specialized areas of sensory epithelium called maculae, which are innervated by fibers of the vestibular division of the vestibulocochlear nerve. These receptors respond to linear acceleration and the static pull of gravity.

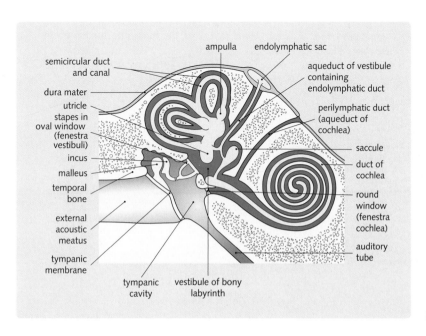

Fig. 8.40 Internal ear.

Semicircular ducts
Within the ampulla of each duct is a sensory area called the ampullary crest, each of which is innervated by the vestibulocochlear nerve. These contain receptors that respond to rotational acceleration in three different planes.

Endolymphatic duct
This duct opens into the endolymphatic sac under the dura mater of the posterior cranial fossa. The sac is a storage reservoir for excess endolymph.

Vestibulocochlear nerve (VIII)
CN VIII emerges from the junction of the pons and medulla, and enters the internal auditory meatus, where it divides into an anterior cochlear nerve (hearing) and a posterior vestibular nerve (balance), as shown in Fig. 8.41. The vestibular nerve contains axons of neurons with nerve cell bodies in the vestibular ganglion, and its fibers supply receptors in the ampullae of the semicircular ducts and the maculae of the saccule and the utricle. The cochlear nerve is formed from the fibers of nerves with cell bodies in the spiral ganglion and supplies the spiral organ.

Facial nerve in the temporal bone
The facial nerve (CN VII) and its sensory root—the nervus intermedius—also emerge from the junction of the pons and medulla and enter the internal auditory meatus together with the VIII nerve. The two roots fuse and enter the facial canal to pass above the internal ear to reach the medial wall of the middle ear. The nerve then makes a sharp posterior turn above the promontory. The sensory geniculate ganglion lies at the sharp bend that the nerve makes on entering the middle ear. It then passes posteriorly to the posterior wall of the tympanic cavity, where it turns downwards to leave the temporal bone through the stylomastoid foramen.

Branches in the temporal bone
Branches within the facial canal of the temporal bone are:
- The greater petrosal nerve, which carries sensory fibers. This branches off at the geniculate ganglion and runs forward through the petrosal bone to enter the middle cranial fossa. It is joined by the deep petrosal nerve to form the nerve of the pterygoid canal.
- The nerve to stapedius.
- The chorda tympani. This is given off just above the stylomastoid foramen. It passes to the lateral wall of the middle ear, crosses the deep surface of the tympanic membrane, and enters a canal leading to the petrotympanic fissure. It joins the lingual nerve in the infratemporal fossa.

The soft tissues of the neck

The neck is the region between the head and the thorax.

Fascial layers of the neck
The fascial layers of the neck are illustrated in Fig. 8.42.

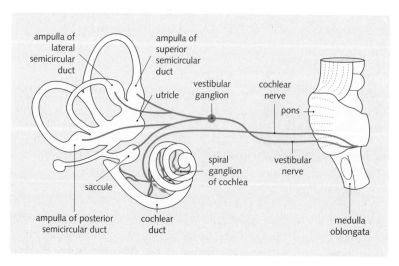

Fig. 8.41 Vestibulocochlear nerve.

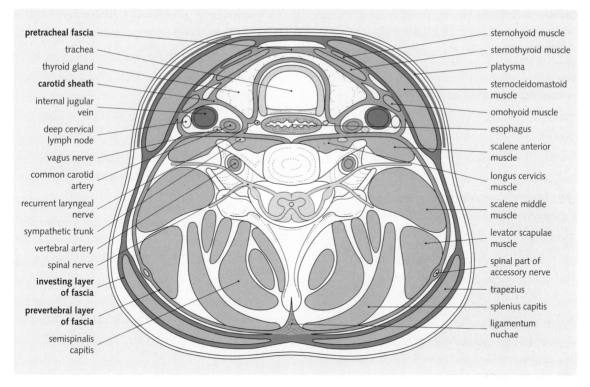

Fig. 8.42 Fascial layers of the neck.

Superficial fascia

The superficial fascia is a thin layer between the dermis and the deep fascia. Anterolaterally, it encloses the platysma muscle. The cutaneous nerves, superficial vessels, and superficial lymph nodes lie in the fascia.

Deep fascia

The deep fascia lies beneath the superficial fascia. It can be subdivided into four regional layers: an investing layer of deep cervical fascia, the pretracheal fascia, the prevertebral fascia, and the carotid sheath. These layers form cleavage planes between the structures they invest, which can be separated during surgery. They also limit the spread of infection.

Investing layer of deep cervical fascia

This completely encircles the neck, splitting to enclose the sternocleidomastoid and trapezius muscles. Superiorly, it is attached to the superior nuchal line of the occipital bone, the mastoid process of the temporal bone, the zygomatic arch, the inferior border of the mandible, the hyoid

bone, and the spinous processes of the cervical vertebrae. It splits to enclose the submandibular gland and the parotid gland. The stylomandibular ligament is a thickening of the fascia between the angle of the mandible and the styloid process.

Inferiorly, the fascia is attached to the acromion and spine of the scapula, the clavicle, and the manubrium. It attaches to the anterior and posterior borders of the manubrium to form the suprasternal space, which contains the jugular arch.

Pretracheal fascia

The pretracheal fascia is attached superiorly to the hyoid bone. Inferiorly, it enters the thorax to blend with the fibrous pericardium. Laterally, it blends with the carotid sheath. It encloses the thyroid gland and the parathyroid glands, the trachea, esophagus, and the infrahyoid muscles.

Prevertebral fascia

This fascia is a sheath for the vertebral column and its associated muscles (longus capitis, longus colli, scalene muscles), and it is attached posteriorly to the ligamentum nuchae. It forms the floor of the posterior triangle. Laterally, it forms the axillary sheath, which surrounds the axillary artery and the brachial plexus. Superiorly, it is attached to the base of the skull and inferiorly, it enters the thorax to fuse with the anterior longitudinal ligament of the vertebral column at the level of T3. The retropharyngeal space lies between the prevertebral fascia and the pharynx and esophagus.

> Abscess formation behind the prevertebral fascia can extend laterally in the neck, forming a swelling posterior to the sternocleidomastoid muscle. If it pierces the fascia anteriorly it enters the retropharyngeal space and can narrow the pharynx, causing swallowing (dysphagia) and speaking (disarthria) difficulties.

Carotid sheath
The carotid sheath is a condensation of the fascia surrounding the common and internal carotid arteries, sympathetic nerve fibers, the internal jugular vein, the deep cervical chain of nodes, and the vagus nerve. It extends from the base of the skull to the root of the neck, and it blends with the investing and pretracheal fascia anteriorly and the prevertebral fascia posteriorly.

Posterior triangle of the neck
The margins and contents of the posterior triangle are detailed in Figs. 8.43 and 8.44, respectively.

Margins of the posterior triangle	
Margin	Components
Anterior	Posterior border of sternomastoid
Posterior	Anterior border of trapezius
Inferior	Middle third of clavicle
Roof	Skin, superficial fascia, platysma, investing layer of deep fascia
Floor	Prevertebral fascia covering muscles of floor

Fig. 8.43 Margins of the posterior triangle.

The inferior belly of omohyoid divides the posterior triangle into a large occipital triangle and a small supraclavicular triangle (Fig. 8.45).

Fig. 8.46 outlines the muscles on the lateral aspect of the neck.

Cervical plexus
The cervical plexus is formed by the anterior rami of C1–C4 spinal nerves. Cervical nerves 2–4 divide into ascending and descending branches, which unite with branches of adjacent nerves to form loops. The loops and branches of the loops comprise the cervical plexus and lie anterolaterally to the levator scapulae and middle scalene muscles (Fig. 8.47).

The ansa cervicalis is a loop formed from an inferior root, which is a branch of the cervical plexus (typically C2 and C3), and a superior root that is formed from fibers from C1 and C2 spinal nerves, which travel with the hypoglossal nerve for a short distance. The inferior and superior roots meet in a loop either around the internal jugular vein or deep to it, and branches from this loop innervate the infrahyoid muscles.

Contents of the posterior triangle	
Structure	Origin
Third part of sublcavian artery	Enters anteroinferior angle of triangle
Part of external jugular vein	Enters anteroinferior part of triangle through the deep fascia
Transverse cervical artery	Branch of thyrocervical trunk of subclavian artery
Suprascapular artery	Branch of thyrocervical trunk
Brachial plexus	Roots of plexus enter posteior triangle by emerging between anterior and middle scalene muscles; trunks and divisions also lie in posterior triangle before entering the axilla
Accessory nerve	Spinal part of accessory nerve enters posterior triangle by emerging from deep to posterior border of sternocleidomastoid
Cervical plexus	The four cutaneous branches emerge from posterior border of sternocleidomastoid

Fig. 8.44 Contents of the posterior triangle.

Fig. 8.45 Posterior triangle of the neck.

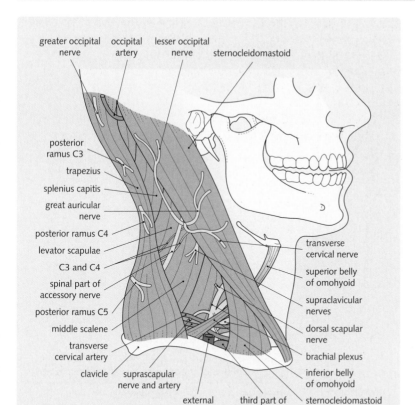

greater occipital nerve
occipital artery
lesser occipital nerve
sternocleidomastoid

posterior ramus C3
trapezius
splenius capitis
great auricular nerve
posterior ramus C4
levator scapulae
C3 and C4
spinal part of accessory nerve
posterior ramus C5
middle scalene
transverse cervical artery
clavicle
suprascapular nerve and artery

transverse cervical nerve
superior belly of omohyoid
supraclavicular nerves
dorsal scapular nerve
brachial plexus
inferior belly of omohyoid
sternocleidomastoid

external jugular vein
third part of subclavian artery

Fig. 8.46 Major muscles of the lateral aspect of the neck.

Major muscles of the lateral aspect of the neck			
Name of muscle	**Superior attachment**	**Inferior attachment**	**Action**
Platysma (CNII)	Inferior border of mandible; skin and subcutaneous tissues of lower part of the face	Fascia covering superior parts of pectoralis major and deltoid muscles	Used to express sadness and fright by pulling down angles of mouth
Sternocleidomastoid (CNXI [spinal part], C2, C3)	Lateral surface of mastoid process of temporal bone and lateral superior nuchal line	Anterior surface of manubrium of sternum; superior surface of medial third of clavicle	Individually each muscle laterally flexes neck and rotates it so that face is turned upward toward opposite side; both muscles act together to flex neck
Trapezius (CNXI [spinal part], C3, C4)	Superior nuchal line; external occipital protuberance; ligamentum nuchae; spinous processes of C7–T12 vertebrae	Lateral third of clavicle; acromion; spine of scapula	Elevates, retracts, and rotates scapula

Fig. 8.46 Major muscles of the lateral aspect of the neck.

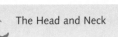

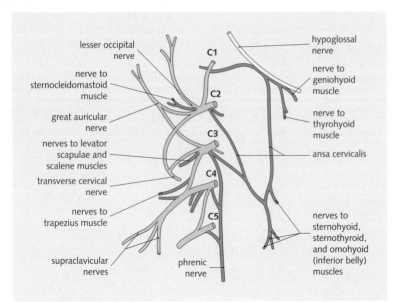

Fig. 8.47 Branches of the cervical plexus.

Labels in figure:
- lesser occipital nerve
- C1
- hypoglossal nerve
- nerve to sternocleidomastoid muscle
- C2
- nerve to geniohyoid muscle
- great auricular nerve
- C3
- nerve to thyrohyoid muscle
- nerves to levator scapulae and scalene muscles
- ansa cervicalis
- transverse cervical nerve
- C4
- nerves to trapezius muscle
- C5
- supraclavicular nerves
- phrenic nerve
- nerves to sternohyoid, sternothyroid, and omohyoid (inferior belly) muscles

External jugular vein

The external jugular vein is formed by the union of the posterior auricular vein and the posterior division of the retromandibular vein behind the angle of the mandible. It crosses the sternocleidomastoid muscle deep to the platysma and pierces the deep fascia just above the clavicle in the posterior triangle to enter the subclavian vein.

Anterior triangle of the neck

The anterior triangle is formed by the anterior border of sternocleidomastoid muscle posteriorly, the midline of the neck anteriorly, and the inferior border of the mandible superiorly. It is subdivided by the anterior and posterior bellies of digastric and the superior belly of omohyoid into the submandibular (digastric), carotid, and muscular triangles and an unpaired submental triangle (Figs. 8.48 and 8.49).

The boundaries of these triangles are as follows:
- Carotid triangle: anterior border of sternocleidomastoid, posterior belly of digastric, superior belly of omohyoid muscles.
- Submandibular (or digastric) triangle: inferior border of mandible, anterior and posterior bellies of digastric muscle.
- Submental (below chin) triangle: body of hyoid bone and anterior bellies of the right and left digastric muscles.

Contents of the anterior triangle of the neck	
Triangle	**Main contents**
Carotid	Common carotid artery dividing into internal and external carotids, branches of external carotid, internal jugular vein and its tributaries, vagus nerve, hypoglossal nerve, internal and external laryngeal nerves, deep cervical lymph nodes
Muscular	Sternothyroid, sternohyoid, and thyrohyoid muscles, superior belly of omohyoid; thyroid and parathyroid glands, trachea, and esophagus
Digastric (submandibular)	Submandibular gland and lymph nodes; facial artery and vein; external carotid artery; internal carotid artery; internal jugular vein; glossopharyngeal (IX), vagus (X), and hypoglossal (XII) nerves
Submental	Submental lymph nodes

Fig. 8.48 Contents of the anterior triangle of the neck.

- Muscular triangle: hyoid bone, anterior border of the sternocleidomastoid, superior belly of omohyoid muscle, and median plane of the neck.

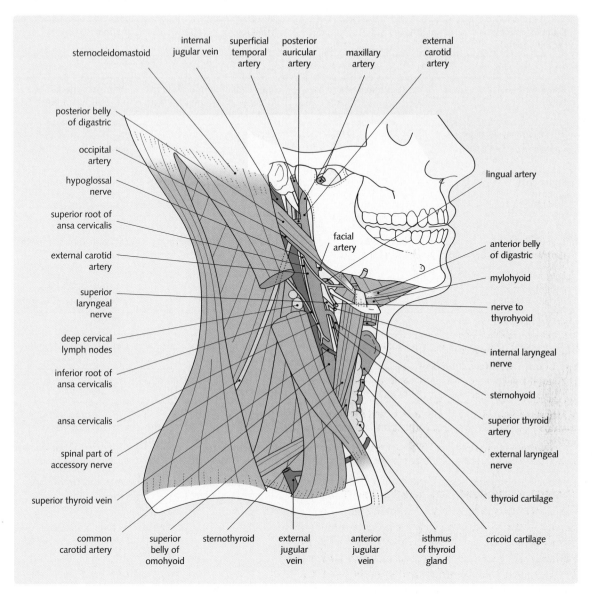

Fig. 8.49 Anterior triangle of the neck.

The muscles of the anterior triangle are shown in Fig. 8.50, and the contents are detailed in Figs. 8.48 and 8.49.

Vessels of the anterior triangle
Common carotid artery

The left common carotid artery arises from the aortic arch, the right from the brachiocephalic trunk. Both ascend in the neck deep to the sternocleidomastoid muscle behind the sternoclavicular joint. At the level of the upper border of the thyroid cartilage the arteries divide into the external and internal carotid arteries (Fig. 8.51).

At the terminal part of the common carotid artery and the origin of the internal carotid artery there is a localized dilatation, the carotid sinus. The sinus contains baroreceptors that respond to increases in arterial pressure, reflexively lowering the pressure.

The carotid body lies at the bifurcation of the common carotid, embedded in the tunica

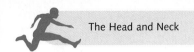
Suprahyoid and infrahyoid muscles			
Name of muscle (nerve supply)	**Origin**	**Insertion**	**Action**
Suprahyoid muscles			
Posterior belly of digastric (CNVII)	Mastoid notch of temporal bone	Intermediate tendon bound to body and greater horn of hyoid bone	Depresses mandible and elevates hyoid bone
Anterior belly of disgastric (inferior alveolar/CNV₃)	Digastric fossa of mandible	Intermediate tendon bound to body and greater horn of hyoid bone	Depresses mandible and elevates hyoid bone
Stylohyoid (CNVII)	Styloid process of temporal bone	Body of hyoid bone	Elevates and retracts hyoid bone and elongates floor of mouth
Mylohyoid (inferior alveolar/CNV₃)	Mylohyoid line on medial surface of mandible	Body of hyoid bone and mylohyoid raphe	Elevates floor of mouth and tongue during swallowing and speech
Geniohyoid (C1 via CNXII)	Inferior mental spine	Body of hyoid bone	Elevates hyoid bone and shortens floor of mouth
Infrahyoid muscles			
Sternohyoid (ansa cervicalis C1–C3)	Manubrium of sternum and medial end of clavicle	Body of hyoid bone	Depresses hyoid bone after swallowing
Sternothyroid (ansa cervicalis C1–C3)	Posterior surface of manubrium of sternum	Oblique line on lamina of thyroid cartilage	Depresses hyoid bone and larynx
Thyrohoid (C1 via CNXII)	Oblique line on lamina of thyroid cartilage	Body of hyoid bone	Depresses hyoid bone and elevates larynx
Omohyoid—inferior belly (ansa cervicalis C1–C3)	Superior margin of scapula near suprascapular notch	Intermediate tendon bound to clavicle and first rib	Depresses, retracts, and steadies hyoid bone
Omohyoid—superior belly (ansa cervicalis C1–C3)	Inferior border of body of hyoid bone	Intermediate tendon bound to clavicle and first rib	Depresses hyoid bone

Fig. 8.50 Suprahyoid and infrahyoid muscles.

adventitia. It contains chemoreceptors that monitor reduced oxygen levels in the blood, reflexively increasing the depth and rapidity of breathing. It also reacts to changes in head position and gravity to maintain the flow of blood to the brain.

Both the carotid sinus and the carotid body are innervated by the carotid sinus branch of CN IX nerve.

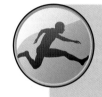

The common carotid pulse can be palpated at the upper border of the thyroid cartilage (C3, C4 vertebral levels), anterior to the sternocleidomastoid muscle.

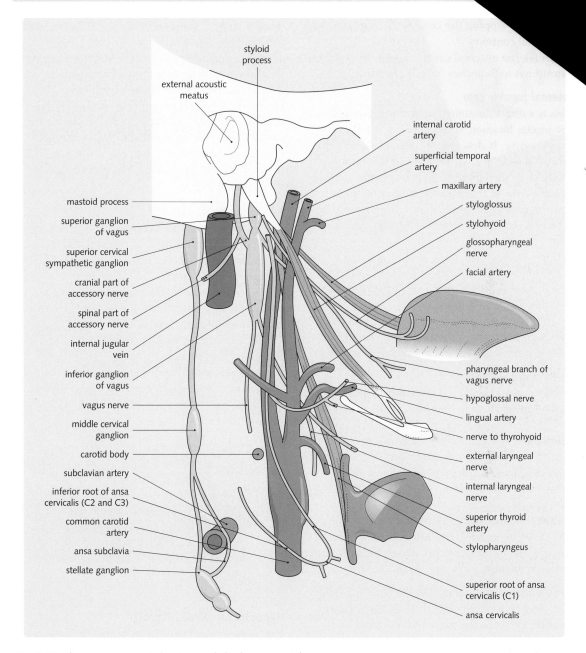

Fig. 8.51 The common carotid artery and the lower cranial nerves.

External carotid artery

This commences at the upper border of the thyroid cartilage and ascends to enter the parotid. Eight main branches supply most of the head except for the brain and orbit and help supply the neck:

- Ascending pharyngeal.
- Superior thyroid.
- Lingual.
- Facial.
- Occipital.
- Posterior auricular.
- Superficial temporal.
- Maxillary.

Internal carotid artery

This commences at the upper border of the thyroid cartilage, and it ascends in the carotid sheath deep to the mandible to the carotid canal in the base of

207

...bral hemispheres and

...otid artery, the internal
...utside the skull.

...tion of the sigmoid sinus at
...rough which it leaves the
cranial ca... ...ends through the neck in the
carotid sheath, a... ...t posterior to the carotid
artery and then lateral to it. It leaves the anterior
triangle deep to the sternocleidomastoid muscle
and unites with the subclavian vein to form the
brachiocephalic vein behind the sternoclavicular
joint.

The vein has dilatations at its upper and lower
ends—the superior and inferior bulbs, respectively.
The inferior bulb contains a valve that prevents
backflow of blood into the vein.

Tributaries include the inferior petrosal sinus,
the facial vein, the pharyngeal vein, the lingual
vein, and the superior and middle thyroid veins.

Deep cervical nodes

These form a chain along the internal jugular vein
in the carotid sheath. They directly or indirectly
drain the entire head and neck region. Efferent
vessels join to form the jugular lymph trunk, which
in turn drains into the thoracic duct, or, on the
right side, into the right lymph duct or the
subclavian trunk (see Fig. 8.12).

Nerves of the triangles of the neck

The following nerves are all found in the anterior
triangle except the accessory nerve, which is in the
posterior triangle.

Glossopharyngeal nerve (CN IX)

This nerve leaves the skull through the jugular
foramen between the two carotid arteries and
passes between the superior and middle
constrictors to supply sensory and taste fibers to
the posterior third of the tongue and sensory fibers
to the pharynx, palatine tonsil, soft palate,
posterior third of the tongue, auditory tube, and
carotid sinus and body. Its motor branch supplies
the stylopharyngeus muscle. It carries
parasympathetic fibers to the parotid gland.

Vagus nerve (CN X)

The vagus arises from the medulla and exits the
skull through the jugular foramen. It has a superior
sensory ganglion in the jugular foramen and an
inferior sensory ganglion below the foramen. Below
the superior ganglion the cranial part of the
accessory nerve joins the vagus, and its fibers are
distributed with the branches of the vagus to the
soft palate, pharynx, esophagus, and larynx
(recurrent laryngeal nerve) (Fig. 8.52). CN X
descends through the neck in the carotid sheath,
initially between the internal carotid artery and
internal jugular vein. At the root of the neck the
nerve passes anterior to the first part of the
subclavian artery to enter the thorax.

Accessory nerve (CN XI)

The spinal part of the accessory nerve arises from
the upper five or six cervical segments. The roots
ascend in the vertebral canal and enter the skull via
the foramen magnum.

The cranial root arises from the medulla
oblongata. The two roots unite as they exit the
skull via the jugular foramen.

The cranial root immediately joins the vagus;
the spinal root separates to supply the
sternocleidomastoid and then crosses the floor of
the posterior triangle to innervate the trapezius.

Remember that CN XI supplies
the trapezius and
sternocleidomastoid. If CN XI
is damaged, patients cannot
shrug their shoulders or turn
their head against resistance.

Hypoglossal nerve (CN XII)

This nerve arises from the medulla and leaves the
skull via the hypoglossal canal. It descends through
the neck between the internal carotid artery and
the internal jugular vein. At the lower border
of the digastric muscle, the nerve crosses the
internal and external carotid arteries to enter the
submandibular region. It is motor to the muscles of
the tongue.

The XII nerve is joined by fibers of the C1 and
C2 spinal nerves, which then travel with the
hypoglossal for a short distance before leaving to
form the superior root of the ansa cervicalis, as
described previously.

Branches of the vagus nerve	
Branch	**Course and distribution**
Meningeal branch	Dura mater of posterior cranial fossa
Auricular branch	External auditory meatus and adjacent tympanic membrane
Pharyngeal branches	Contain some motor fibers from CNXI (cranial part); also combine with pharyngeal branches of CNIX (sensory fibers) to form pharyngeal plexus; vagal contribution supplies all pharyngeal muscles except stylopharyngeus (IX) and all soft palate muscles except tensor veli palatini (V₃)
Superior laryngeal nerve	Arises from the inferior ganglion of the vagus, descends to the level of the hyoid bone, and divides into internal and external branches. Internal laryngeal branch is sensory to piriform fossa and mucosa of larynx above vocal folds; external laryngeal branch is motor to cricothyroid muscle and inferior pharyngeal contrictor
Cardiac branches	Given off in lower neck, run behind subclavian artery to contribute to cardiac plexus in thorax
Right recurrent laryngeal nerve	Arises from CNX as it crosses subclavian artery; hooks posteriorly and superiorly behind artery and ascends in a groove between trachea and esophagus; supplies trachea and esophagus and ends as inferior laryngeal nerve to all laryngeal muscles (except cricothyroid) and laryngeal mucosa below vocal fold
Left recurrent laryngeal	Arises from CNX as it crosses aortic arch, hooks beneath arch and inferior to ligamentum arteriosum and passes into neck between trachea and esophagus; has a similar distribution to right nerve

Fig. 8.52 Branches of the vagus nerve.

Sympathetic trunk

The sympathetic trunk in the neck lies anterolateral to the vertebral column. This trunk receives no white rami communicantes, but has superior, middle, and inferior ganglia. The ganglia receive presynaptic fibers from the superior thoracic spinal nerves via white rami communicantes to the thoracic sympathetic trunk. The inferior ganglion usually fuses with the first thoracic ganglion to form the stellate ganglion anterior to the transverse process of the C7 vertebra. Postganglionic fibers form plexuses around the major vessels, especially the vertebral and internal and external carotid arteries, and supply the structures of the head and neck (e.g., blood vessels and glands). They also pass to the cervical spinal nerves via gray rami communicantes, and a splanchnic nerve, the inferior cervical cardiac nerve, passes to the cardiac plexus of the heart.

A cervical sympathetic trunk lesion results in ipsilateral papillary constriction, ptosis (drooping of the upper eyelid), facial and neck vasodilation, lack of sweating, and sinking in of the eye. This is due to an interrupted sympathetic nerve supply; it is called Horner's syndrome.

209

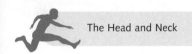

Midline structures of the face and neck

Pharynx

The pharynx is a fibromuscular tube that can be subdivided into three regions:

- The nasopharynx—posterior to the nasal cavity.
- The oropharynx—posterior to the oral cavity.
- The laryngopharynx—posterior to the larynx.

It extends from the base of the skull to the inferior border of the cricoid cartilage (C6 vertebra level), where it is continuous with the esophagus. There are three layers in the pharyngeal wall, from external to internal:

- The muscular layer is formed by the pharyngeal constrictors and longitudinal muscles (Figs. 8.53 and 8.54).
- The pharyngobasilar fascia is the strong lining internal to the pharyngeal constrictors. It blends with the pretracheal fascia of the deep cervical fascia inferiorly.
- The mucous membrane (Fig. 8.55).

Nasopharynx

The nasopharynx is a posterior extension of the nasal cavity. Anteriorly, it is continuous with the nose through paired openings called choanae, and it lies above the soft palate. The roof is mucous membrane applied to the basal portions of the sphenoid and occipital bones. On the lateral walls, above the soft palate, are the ostia of the auditory tubes. An elevation above each ostium, created by the protruding cartilage of the tube, is called the torus tubarius. The pharyngeal recess is a slit-like opening in the lateral wall behind the torus.

Lymphoid tissue is aggregated in regions of the nasopharynx to form tonsils. The pharyngeal tonsil lies in the mucous membrane of the roof and posterior wall. Tubal tonsils are found adjacent to the ostia of the auditory tubes.

During deglutition (swallowing), the soft palate elevates and the pharyngeal wall is pulled forward to form a seal, preventing food entering the nasopharynx.

\multicolumn{4}{c}{Muscles of the pharynx}
Name of muscle (nerve supply)	Origin	Insertion	Action
Superior constrictor (pharyngeal plexus)	Pterygoid hamulus, pterygomandibular raphe, posterior end of hylohyoid line of mandible, side of tongue	Pharyngeal tubercle of occipital bone, midline pharyngeal raphe	Initiates progressive constriction of pharynx and propels food bolus downward during swallowing
Middle contrictor (pharyngeal plexus)	Stylohyoid ligament, lesser and greater cornua of hyoid bone	Pharyngeal raphe	Constriction of pharynx during swallowing propels food bolus downward
Inferior constrictor (pharyngeal plexus)	Oblique line of lamina of of thyroid cartilage and side of cricoid cartilage (cricopharyngeus)	Pharyngeal raphe; contralateral cricopharyngeus	Constriction of pharynx during swallowing propels food bolus downward; sphincter at inferior end of pharynx (cricopharyngeus)
Palatopharyngeus (pharyngeal plexus)	Palantine aponeurosis Horizontal plate of palatine bone	Posterior lamina of thyroid cartilage	Elevates pharyngeal wall and pulls palatopharyngeal arch medially
Salpingopharyngeus (pharyngeal plexus)	Cartilagenous part of auditory tube	Merges with palatopharyngeus	Elevates pharynx and larynx during swallowing and speech
Stylopharyngeus (CNIX)	Styloid process of temporal bone	Posterior and superior borders of thyroid cartilage	Elevates larynx during swallowing and speech

Fig. 8.53 Muscles of the pharynx.

Fig. 8.54 Muscles of the pharynx.

pterygomandibular raphe

pterygoid hamulus

medial pterygoid plate

opening for auditory tube

pharyngobasilar fascia

superior pharyngeal constrictor muscle

stylopharyngeus muscle

middle pharyngeal constrictor muscle

superior laryngeal artery, nerve, and vein

inferior pharyngeal constrictor muscle

stylohyoid ligament

hyoid bone

thyroid cartilage

oblique line

cricoid cartilage

cricopharyngeal part of inferior pharyngeal constrictor muscle

esophagus

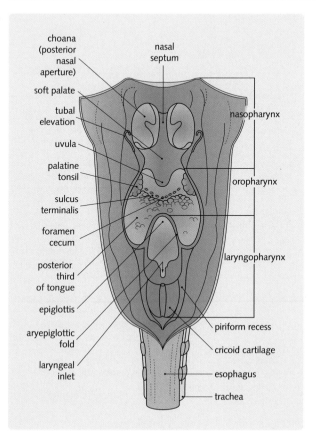

choana (posterior nasal aperture)

nasal septum

soft palate

nasopharynx

tubal elevation

uvula

palatine tonsil

oropharynx

sulcus terminalis

foramen cecum

posterior third of tongue

laryngopharynx

epiglottis

aryepiglottic fold

piriform recess

laryngeal inlet

cricoid cartilage

esophagus

trachea

Fig. 8.55 Mucous membrane and the interior of the pharynx, posterior view.

Pharyngeal mucosa can bulge between the thyropharyngeus and cricopharyngeal muscles to form a pharyngeal pouch (Killian's dehiscence).

Oropharynx

The oropharynx extends from the soft palate superiorly to the upper border of the epiglottis inferiorly. The lateral walls of the oropharynx each have two folds of mucosa—an anterior palatoglossal fold over palatoglossus muscle and a posteriorly palatopharyngeal fold over the palatopharyngeus muscle. The palatoglossal arch, formed by the folds on either side, marks the boundary between the mouth and the oropharynx. The palatine tonsils lie in the recesses between these two folds on either side. The anterior wall of the oropharynx is formed by the posterior third of the tongue. It has an irregular surface owing to the presence of the underlying lingual tonsils.

The mucosa is reflected from the tongue onto the epiglottis to form a median and two lateral glossoepiglottic folds. The depression on each side of the median fold is the vallecula.

Laryngopharynx

The laryngopharynx extends from the superior border of the epiglottis and laryngeal inlet to the level of the inferior border of the cricoid cartilage. Here it narrows and becomes continuous with the esophagus.

The piriform recesses are grooves on either side of the laryngeal inlet, separated from the inlet by the aryepiglottic folds.

Vessels of the pharynx

Blood supply to the pharynx is from branches of the ascending pharyngeal, ascending palatine, and lingual arteries, and the tonsillary artery, a branch of the facial.

Veins drain via the pharyngeal venous plexus to the internal jugular vein.

Lymphatics drain into the deep cervical nodes either directly or indirectly via the retropharyngeal or paratracheal nodes.

Nerve supply of the pharynx

The motor nerve supply to the pharynx is the cranial part of CN XI via CN X and the pharyngeal plexus.

The sensory nerve supply is as follows:
- Nasopharynx—maxillary nerve (CN V_2).
- Oropharynx—CN IX.
- Laryngopharynx—internal laryngeal nerve (branch of CN X).

Nose

The nose consists of:
- The external nose—this has a bony (nasal bones, frontal process of the maxilla, nasal part of the frontal bone) and cartilaginous skeleton (alar and lateral cartilages), separated by the nasal septum, which is also both bony and cartilaginous (Fig. 8.56).
- The nasal cavities—these communicate with the exterior via the nares or nostrils anteriorly, and with the nasopharynx via the choanae posteriorly.

Walls of the nasal cavity	
Surface	**Components**
Floor	Palatine process of maxilla, horizontal process of palatine bone—i.e., the hard palate
Roof	Nasal, frontal, sphenoid, and ethmoid bones; above lies the anterior cranial fossa and the sphenoid sinus
Lateral wall	Frontal process of maxilla, palatine, sphenoid, lacrimal, nasal, and ethmoid bones and the inferior concha; the superior and middle conchae are projections of the ethmoid bone; beneath the three conchae are the superior, middle, and inferior meati, respectively, and the sphenoethmoidal recess above the superior concha
Medial wall (nasal septum)	The perpendicular plate of the ethmoid, the vomer, and the septal cartilage

Fig. 8.56 Walls of the nasal cavity.

Features and openings in the lateral wall of the nose	
Region of lateral wall	Features and openings
Sphenoethmoidal recess	Sphenoidal sinus
Superior meatus	Posterior ethmoidal air cells
Middle meatus	Hiatus semilunaris (a semicircular groove below the conchae)—frontal sinus anteriorly, maxillary sinus posteriorly, anterior ethmoid air cells Ethmoid bulla (rounded prominence above the hiatus)—middle ethmoid air cells
Inferior meatus	Nasolacrimal duct anteriorly

Fig. 8.57 Features and openings in the lateral wall of the nose.

Nasal cavity

The composition of the walls of the nasal cavity is described in Fig. 8.56. Of particular note are three scroll-shaped projections on the lateral wall—the superior, middle, and inferior conchae. Below each concha is a recess called a meatus. Above the superior concha is the sphenoethmoidal recess.

The openings in the lateral wall are listed in Fig. 8.57.

The nerve and blood supply of the lateral wall are illustrated in Fig. 8.58.

Fractures of the nasal bones are a common sports injury. If the injury results from a direct blow (punch or elbow to the nose), the cribiform plate of the ethmoid bone may also fracture, and the cranial meninges can be torn, allowing bacteria from the nasal cavity to enter the cranial cavity.

Paranasal sinuses

The paranasal sinuses are air-filled extensions of the respiratory portion of the nasal cavity, in the bones of the face and skull. They are named for those bones: the sphenoidal, ethmoidal, frontal, and maxillary sinuses. They drain into the nasal cavity.

Mucous membrane of the nose

The vestibule lies just inside the anterior nares and is lined by hairy skin. The remainder of the nasal

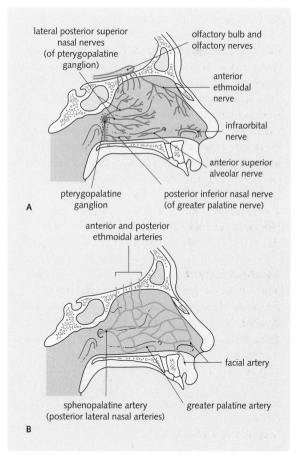

Fig. 8.58 Nerve (A) and blood (B) supplies of the lateral wall of the nose.

cavity is lined by ciliated columnar epithelium. There is a rich vascular plexus in the submucosa, together with numerous serous and mucous glands. The inferior two-thirds of the nasal mucosa is the

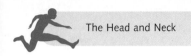

respiratory area, while the superior one-third is olfactory.

Dust from the inspired air is removed by the nasal hairs and the mucus of the nasal cavity. The air is also warmed by the vascular plexus and moistened before it enters the lower airway.

The roof and superior part of the lateral wall contain olfactory epithelium, which receives dendrites of the olfactory nerve cells in the olfactory bulbs, lying above the roof (cribriform plate). These fibers carry both smell and taste information.

The sphenopalatine artery anastomoses with the septal branch of the superior labial artery around the vestibule of the nose. This is a very common site for a nosebleed (epistaxis).

Pterygopalatine fossa

The pterygopalatine fossa is a small but important pyramidal space lying inferior to the apex of the orbit. It lies between the maxilla anteriorly and the pterygoid process of the sphenoid bone posteriorly. It contains the terminal branches of the maxillary artery, the maxillary nerve, the nerve of the pterygoid canal, and the pterygopalatine ganglion. The communications of the fossa are listed in Fig. 8.59.

Pterygopalatine ganglion

The pterygopalatine ganglion is a parasympathetic ganglion lying in the superior pterygopalatine fossa, suspended from the maxillary nerve (V_2) by two pterygopalatine nerves.

Preganglionic parasympathetic fibers from the superior salivary nucleus of CN VII form the greater petrosal nerve that arises at the geniculate ganglion and passes through the petrous ridge of the temporal bone to join the deep petrosal (sympathetic) nerve from the external carotid plexus. They form the nerve of the pterygoid canal. This nerve traverses the pterygoid canal to join the ganglion. Here, the parasympathetic fibers synapse and sympathetic fibers pass uninterrupted through the ganglion. Sensory fibers of V_2 enter the ganglion via the pterygopalatine nerves.

The branches of the ganglion are shown in Fig. 8.60.

Oral cavity

The oral cavity is divided into the oral vestibule and the oral cavity proper.

The vestibule is a slit-like space between the lips and cheeks externally and the gums (buccal gingiva) and teeth internally.

The oral cavity proper is bounded by dental arches anteriorly and laterally. The palate forms the roof; the floor is formed by the anterior two-thirds of the tongue and the floor of the mouth. A midline fold of mucosa—the frenulum—runs on the floor of the mouth to the posterioinferior surface of the tongue (Fig. 8.61). Posteriorly it communicates with the oropharynx.

The submandibular ducts open onto the sublingual papillae on either side of the frenulum. The sublingual fold extends back from the papilla and overlies the sublingual glands. Numerous small ducts from these glands open onto the folds. Opposite the upper second molar on the internal surface of each cheek is the opening of the parotid duct from the parotid gland.

Nerve supply is as follows:
- Roof—greater and lesser palatine and nasopalatine nerves.
- Floor—lingual nerve.
- Cheek—buccal nerve (from CN V_3).

Lips

The two lips are muscular folds that seal the oral cavity anteriorly, and they also assist in speech. The lips are covered by mucosa internally and by skin externally. The orbicularis oris muscle, the superior and inferior labial muscles, vessels, and nerves, and numerous minor salivary glands lie in the substance of the lips. The upper lip has a depression called the philtrum that extends to it from the external nasal septum, and the lips are separated from the

Communications of the pterygopalatine fossa	
Surface	**Communicates with**
Lateral	Infratemporal fossa via the pterygomaxillary fissure
Medial	Nasal cavity via the sphenopalatine foramen
Anterior	Orbit via the interior orbital fissure
Posterosuperior	Midline cranial fossa via the foramen rotundum and pterygoid canal

Fig. 8.59 Communications of the pterygopalatine fossa.

Branches of the pterygopalatine ganglion	
Branch	**Course and distribtuion**
Nasopalatine nerve	Passses through the sphenopalatine foramen to supply the nasal septum and the hard palate behind the incisor teeth
Lateral posterior superior nasal nerve	Exits via the sphenopalatine foramen to supply the lateral wall of the nose
Greater palatine nerve	Passes through the greater palatine foramina to the greater palatine canal to supply the mucosa of the palate and the lateral wall of the nose
Lesser palatine nerve	Exits through the lesser palatine foramina to the lesser palatine canals to supply the soft palate and the mucosa over the palatine tonsil
Pharyngeal nerves	Tiny nerves that pass via the palatovaginal canal to supply the nasopharynx
Lacrimal fibers	Parasympathetic fibers to the lacrimal gland join the zygmaticotemporal nerve of the zygomatic nerve of CNV$_2$, then the lacrimal nerve, before supplying the gland

Fig. 8.60 Branches of the pterygopalatine ganglion.

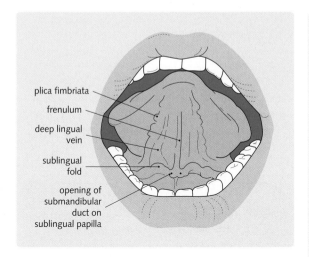

Fig. 8.61 Oral cavity.

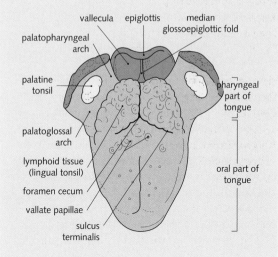

Fig. 8.62 Tongue.

cheeks by the nasolabial folds that extend from the nose to the angles of the mouth.

Tongue

The tongue is a mobile muscular organ covered by mucous membrane. The anterior two-thirds lie in the mouth, the posterior third in the oropharynx (Fig. 8.62).

The muscles of the tongue are listed in Fig. 8.63.

Mucous membrane of the tongue

The sulcus terminalis is a V-shaped groove on the posterosuperior surface of the tongue that divides the tongue into the anterior two-thirds and the posterior third. The foramen cecum is a small pit that lies at the apex of the sulcus. It is the remnant of the upper end of the embryonic thyroglossal

215

Muscles of the tongue			
Name of muscle (nerve supply)	Origin	Insertion	Action
Intrinsic muscles			
Longitudinal (CNXII)	Median fibrous septum, margins and root of tongue	Margins and apex of tongue	Shortens tongue
Transverse (CNXII)	Median fibrous septum	Fibrous margins of tongue	Narrows and elongates tongue
Vertical (CNXII)	Superior surface and borders of tongue	Inferior border of tongue	Flattens and broadens tongue
Extrinsic muscles			
Palatoglossus (pharyngeal plexus)	Palatine aponeurosis of soft palate	Lateral aspect of tongue	Elevates posterior tongue and narrows oropharyngeal isthmus
Genioglossus (CNXII)	Superior meatal spine (genial tubercle) of mandible	Dorsum of tongue, body of hyoid bone	Depresses tongue and draws it anteriorly
Hypoglossus (CNXII)	Body and greater cornu of hyoid bone	Sides and inferior aspect of tongue	Depresses and retracts tongue
Styloglossus (CNXII)	Styloid process of temporal bone and stylohyoid ligament	Sides and inferior aspect of tongue	Retracts tongue, creates trough for swallowing

Fig. 8.63 Muscles of the tongue.

duct. Between 10 and 12 large, flat-topped vallate papillae lie anterior to the sulcus. They are surrounded by pits that contain taste buds.

The mucosa of the anterior two-thirds of the tongue is relatively smooth, and it has numerous filiform (sensory to touch) and fungiform papillae on the dorsal surface. The frenulum connects it to the floor of the mouth. Small lateral folds of mucosa, the foliate papillae that also have taste buds, are seen on the sides of the tongue.

The irregular surface of the posterior third of the tongue is caused by the underlying lingual tonsils. A midline groove on the dorsal surface of the tongue indicates the underlying fibrous lingual septum that divides the tongue into right and left halves.

Blood and nerve supply to the tongue

Vessels of the tongue are the dorsal and deep lingual arteries and veins and the sublingual artery.

Lymphatic drainage is to the deep cervical, the submandibular, and the submental nodes. Carcinoma of the tongue may spread via the lymphatics to both sides of the neck, dramatically worsening its prognosis.

The nerve supply to the tongue is shown in Fig. 8.64.

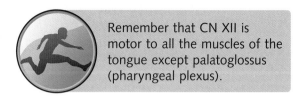

Remember that CN XII is motor to all the muscles of the tongue except palatoglossus (pharyngeal plexus).

Submandibular region

This region lies between the mandible and hyoid bone. It contains the following:

- Muscles—digastric, mylohyoid, hyoglossus, geniohyoid, genioglossus, and styloglossus.
- Salivary glands—submandibular and sublingual.
- Nerves—lingual, glossopharyngeal, and hypoglossal; submandibular ganglion.
- Blood vessels—facial and lingual.
- Lymph nodes—submandibular.

Nerve supply to the tongue		
	Posterior third	**Anterior two-thirds**
General sensory	Glossopharyngeal nerve (CNIX)	Lingual nerve (CNV₃)
Taste	Glossopharyngeal nerve (CNIX) (also vallate papillae)	Chorda tympani (CNVII) (via the lingual nerve)
Motor	Hypoglossal, pharyngeal plexus (palatoglossus) (CNXII, CNXI via CNX)	Hypoglossal nerve (CNXII)

Fig. 8.64 Nerve supply to the tongue.

Submandibular gland

This consists of two parts—a large superficial part above the thyrohyoid muscle and a small deep part below it—that are continuous around the posterior border of mylohyoid. The deep part of the gland lies between the mylohyoid superficially, the styloglossus and hyoglossus inferiorly and medially, and the stylohyoid and anterior belly of the digastric inferiorly and laterally.

Blood supply is from the submental artery from the facial and from the sublingual artery from the lingual artery.

Nerve supply is from the submandibular ganglion, a parasympathetic ganglion with the following features:

• Preganglionic parasympathetic fibers originate in the superior salivary nucleus of the VII nerve and pass to the ganglion via the nervus intermedius, the chorda tympani, and the lingual nerve to synapse in the ganglion.
• Sympathetic and sensory fibers from the superior cervical ganglion and the lingual nerve pass through the ganglion.
• Both postganglionic parasympathetic secretomotor fibers and sympathetic fibers pass to the submandibular and sublingual glands via either the lingual nerve or arteries.

Lingual nerve

This is a branch of V₃. It enters the mouth between the mandible and the medial pterygoid muscle and runs anteriorly under the mucosa. From the mandibular third-molar region, the lingual nerve runs anteriorly on the lateral surface of hyoglossus and across the submandibular duct, to break up into its terminal branches supplying the anterior two-thirds of the tongue and the floor of the mouth.

Hypoglossal nerve

In the submandibular region, the hypoglossal nerve runs forward between the hyoglossus and myelohyoid muscles and below the deep part of the submandibular gland, the submandibular duct, and the lingual nerve. As it curves up toward the tongue, it divides into its terminal branches and supplies all the muscles of the tongue except palatoglossus.

Sublingual gland

The sublingual gland is the smallest of the salivary glands and lies under the mucosa of the floor of the mouth, close to the midline. The lingual nerve and submandibular duct lie medially, the medial surface of the mandible laterally, and the myelohyoid muscle inferiorly. Its nerve supply is the same as that for the submandibular gland.

Palate and tonsils

The palate forms the roof of the mouth and the floor of the nasal cavities. It is divided into two regions:

• Anteriorly, the hard palate is composed of the palatine process of the maxilla and the horizontal process of the palatine bone. The incisive fossa, posterior to the central incisor teeth, has foramina for the nasopalatine nerves. The greater palatine vessels and nerves emerge from the greater palatine foramen on the lateral border of the hard palate, medial to the third molar. Just posterior, the lesser palatine vessels and nerves emerge from the lesser palatine foramen. It is covered by mucous membrane.

• Posteriorly, the soft palate, composed of a mobile fibromuscular fold, extends posteriorly from the hard palate. Within it are muscles (Fig. 8.65) and the palatine aponeurosis—the expanded tendon of tensor veli palatini. From the posterior margin of the soft palate hangs the uvula. When a person swallows, the soft palate tenses to allow the tongue to press against it, forcing food posteriorly.

Blood supply to the palate is from the greater and lesser palatine arteries. Nerve supply is from the pterygopalatine ganglion via greater and lesser palatine nerves and the nasopalatine nerve.

The palatine tonsils are masses of lymphoid tissue lying in the tonsillar fossae between the palatoglossal and palatopharyngeal arches. They are covered by mucous membrane. The surface has many pits that lead into the lymphoid tissue, called tonsillar crypts. Lymphatics drain to the deep cervical nodes.

Larynx

The larynx is continuous with the inferior oropharynx superiorly and with the trachea inferiorly. It acts as a sphincter, separating the lower respiratory system from the alimentary system, and it is responsible for voice production.

The laryngeal cartilages are shown in Fig. 8.66. The laryngeal membranes link these cartilages together, and they join the larynx to the hyoid bone and the trachea inferiorly. The quadrangular membrane is a thin lamina of connective tissue between the thyroid and arytenoid cartilages, which separates the piriform recess from the laryngeal entrance (Fig. 8.67) and supports the aryepiglottic folds. The membranes thicken in places to form ligaments (e.g., the medial and lateral thyrohyoid ligaments in the thyrohyoid membrane).

Arterial and nervous supply to the laryngeal mucosa

Above the vocal fold the mucosa is supplied by the internal laryngeal nerve and the superior laryngeal artery. Below the vocal fold, it is supplied by the recurrent laryngeal nerve and the inferior laryngeal artery (from the inferior thyroid artery).

Laryngeal cavity

The laryngeal inlet allows communication between the oropharynx and the larynx. It is bounded by

Muscles of the soft palate			
Name of muscle (nerve supply)	Origin	Insertion	Action
Tensor veli palatini (nerve to medial pterygoid CNV$_3$)	Spine of sphenoid, cartilage of auditory tube, scaphoid fossa of medial pterygoid plate	With muscle of other side, forms palatine aponeurosis	Tenses soft palate
Levator veli palatini (CNXI via pharyngeal plexus)	Petrous part of temporal bone, cartilage of auditory tube	Palatine aponeurosis	Elevates soft palate
Musculus uvulae (CNXI via pharyngeal plexus)	Posterior border of nasal spine, palatine aponeurosis	Mucous membrane of uvula	Elevates uvula
Palatopharyngeus (CNXI via pharyngeal plexus)	Palatine aponeurosis and horizontal plate of palatine	Posterior border of thyroid cartilage	Tenses soft palate and pulls pharynx superiorly
Palatoglossus (CNXI via pharygeal plexus)	Palatine aponeurosis	Lateral aspect of tongue; lateral wall of pharynx	Pulls tongue upward and backward and draws soft palate onto tongue

Fig. 8.65 Muscles of the soft palate.

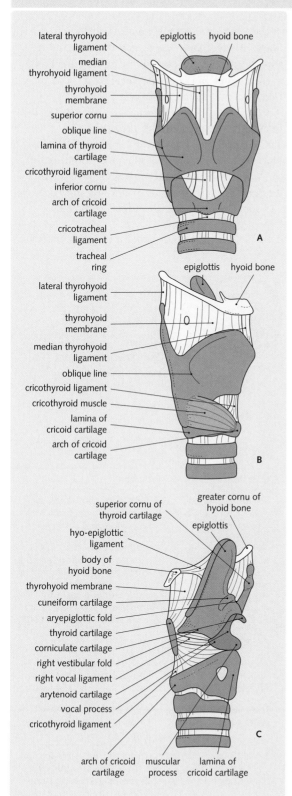

lateral thyrohyoid ligament
epiglottis
hyoid bone
median thyrohyoid ligament
thyrohyoid membrane
superior cornu
oblique line
lamina of thyroid cartilage
cricothyroid ligament
inferior cornu
arch of cricoid cartilage
cricotracheal ligament
tracheal ring
A

epiglottis
hyoid bone
lateral thyrohyoid ligament
thyrohyoid membrane
median thyrohyoid ligament
oblique line
cricothyroid ligament
cricothyroid muscle
lamina of cricoid cartilage
arch of cricoid cartilage
B

superior cornu of thyroid cartilage
greater cornu of hyoid bone
epiglottis
hyo-epiglottic ligament
body of hyoid bone
thyrohyoid membrane
cuneiform cartilage
aryepiglottic fold
thyroid cartilage
corniculate cartilage
right vestibular fold
right vocal ligament
arytenoid cartilage
vocal process
cricothyroid ligament
C

arch of cricoid cartilage
muscular process
lamina of cricoid cartilage

Fig. 8.66 Laryngeal cartilages from the front (A), from the right (B), and from the left without the left lamina of thyroid cartilage (C).

the epiglottis and the aryepiglottic and interarytenoid folds (Fig. 8.68) and can be divided into three regions:

• The vestibule, which extends from the inlet to the vestibular folds.
• The laryngeal ventricle, which lies between the vestibular and vocal folds and which extends anteriorly on either side as small blind sacs—the laryngeal saccules.
• The infraglottic cavity, which extends from the vocal folds superiorly to the trachea inferiorly, at the inferior border of the cricoid cartilage.

The vestibular folds (false vocal folds) consist of two thick folds of mucosa extending between the thyroid and arytenoid cartilages. They contain the vestibular ligament, which is the free edge of the quadrangular ligament.

The vocal folds are wedge-shaped and at their apices is a vocal ligament, consisting of the thickened elastic tissue at the edge of the conus elasticus, a sheet of connective tissue that arises from the upper border of the arch of the cricoid cartilage.

Laryngeal membranes	
Membrane	**Attachment**
Thyrohyoid	Runs between superior border and superior horns of the thyroid cartilage and hyoid bone; has a midline thickening and two lateral thickenings: the medial thyrohyoid ligament and the lateral thyrohyoid ligament, respectively
Quadrangular	Runs between the lateral epiglottic cartilage and the arytenoid cartilage; its lower free border is the vestibular ligament and its upper free edge reinforces the aryepiglottic fold
Cricothyroid	Connects the cricoid cartilage to the lower margin of the thyroid cartilage; it extends superiorly on the deep surface on the thyroid cartilage to which it is attached and where it is called the conus elasticus; its upper free margin forms the vocal ligament
Cricotracheal	Runs from the cricoid cartilage to the trachea

Fig. 8.67 Laryngeal membranes.

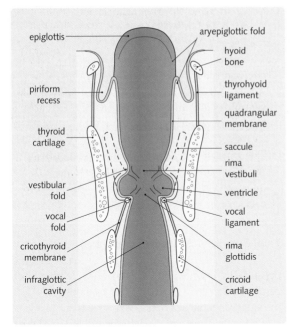

epiglottis

aryepiglottic fold

hyoid bone

thyrohyoid ligament

quadrangular membrane

piriform recess

thyroid cartilage

saccule

rima vestibuli

ventricle

vestibular fold

vocal fold

vocal ligament

cricothyroid membrane

rima glottidis

infraglottic cavity

cricoid cartilage

Fig. 8.68 Coronal section of the laryngeal cavity. (Adapted from Gray's Anatomy 38th edn., edited by L H Bannister et al. Harcourt Brace and Co.)

Also in the vocal folds is the vocalis muscle, the fibers of which are an extension of the thyroarytenoid muscle. The rima glottidis is the narrow space between the vocal folds. The vocal folds are responsible for sound production.

Intrinsic muscles of the larynx

The intrinsic muscles of the larynx are described in Fig. 8.69. All intrinsic muscles are paired except the transverse arytenoid muscle. They alter the tension and length of the vocal folds and the size and shape of the rima glottidis (Fig. 8.70).

All intrinsic muscles are supplied by the recurrent laryngeal nerve except for the cricothyroid muscle, which is supplied by the external laryngeal nerve.

Intrinsic muscles of the larynx			
Muscle (nerve supply)	Origin	Insertion	Action
Cricothyroid (external laryngeal nerve)	Anterolateral cricoid cartilage arch	Inferior border of thyroid cartilage and inferior cornu	Lengthens and tenses vocal cords by tilting cricoid and thus arytenoid cartilages
Posterior cricothyroid (recurrent laryngeal nerve)	Posterior surface of cricoid cartilage lamina	Arytenoid cartilage muscular process	Abducts vocal cords by laterally rotating arytenoid cartilages on cricoid cartilage
Lateral cricothyroid (recurrent laryngeal nerve)	Cricoid cartilage arch	Arytenoid cartilage muscular process	Adducts vocal cords by medially rotating arytenoid cartilage on cricoid cartilage
Thyroarytenoid (recurrent laryngeal nerve)	Posterior surface of thyroid cartilage	Arytenoid cartilage muscular process	Relaxes vocal cord
Transverse arytenoid (recurrent laryngeal nerve)	Body of arytenoid cartilage	Body of opposite arytenoid	Closes rima glottidis by adducting arytenoid cartilage
Oblique arytenoid (recurrent laryngeal nerve)	Muscular process of arytenoid cartilage	Opposite arytenoid cartilage	Closes rima glottidis by drawing arytenoid cartilages together
Vocalis (recurrent laryngeal nerve)	Vocal process of arytenoid cartilage	Vocal ligament	Maintains/increases tension in anterior part of vocal ligament; relaxes posterior part of vocal ligament

Fig. 8.69 Intrinsic muscles of the larynx.

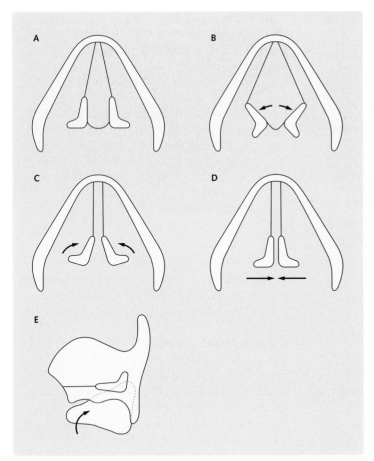

Fig. 8.70 Movements of the vocal folds and arytenoid and cricoid cartilages. (A) Vocal cord position during quiet respiration (i.e., at rest). (B) Vocal cord abduction by posterior cricoarytenoid muscles. (C) Vocal cord adduction by lateral cricoarytenoid muscles. (D) Vocal cord adduction by transverse arytenoid muscle. (E) Increase in vocal cord tension by cricoid cartilage tilting through cricothyroid muscle contraction and drawing arytenoid cartilages posteriorly. (Adapted from Gray's Anatomy 38th edn., edited by L H Bannister et al. Harcourt Brace and Co.)

Joints of the larynx

The synovial cricothyroid joint is formed by the articulation of the inferior cornu (horn) of the thyroid cartilage with the lateral surface of the cricoid cartilage. Around a transverse axis passing through the joints on either side, cricoid cartilages can tilt back and forth on the thyroid cartilage. This alters the vocal fold tension and length.

The synovial cricoarytenoid joint has a lax capsule. This allows rotation and gliding movements of the bases of the arytenoid cartilages on the superolateral surfaces of the laminae of the cricoid cartilage. Arytenoid cartilages can glide toward or away from each other, tilting anteriorly of posteriorly, and can rotate. These movements result in approximating, tensing, and relaxing the vocal folds, which can widen, narrow, or close the V-shaped rima glottidis anteriorly or posteriorly. Thus muscle action on these joints produces changes in the pitch of the voice.

Trachea

The trachea is a fibrocartilagenous tube that commences at the level of C6 vertebra and is continuous with the larynx above. It ends at the sternal angle (T4/T5 vertebral level) by dividing into the right and left main bronchi. Its walls are reinforced by C-shaped hyaline cartilage rings that are deficient posteriorly. The common carotid arteries are related to their lateral aspects.

Thyroid gland

The thyroid gland is a highly vascularized, ductless endocrine gland. It lies anteriorly in the neck, beneath the sternohyoid and sternothyroid muscles, from the C5 to the T1 vertebral levels. It has two lobes connected by a narrow isthmus over the second and third tracheal rings (Fig. 8.71). It regulates the metabolic rate and calcuim metabolism by producing thyroid hormone and calcitonin, respectively.

221

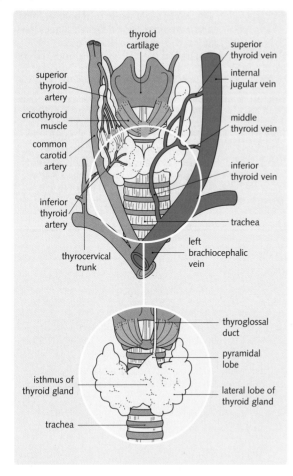

Fig. 8.71 Anterior view of the thyroid gland. The left side of the figure shows the arterial supply, and the right side shows the venous drainage. Inset shows thyroid gland anatomy.

Blood supply to the thyroid gland
The superior thyroid artery (the external carotid artery's first branch) descends to the upper pole of the thyroid with the external laryngeal nerve running with it, and it divides into anterior and posterior branches. The inferior thyroid artery (arising from the thyrocervical trunk of the subclavian artery) runs superomedially before joining the recurrent laryngeal nerve as it reaches the inferior pole of the gland. The inferior artery anastomoses with its superior counterpart.

The thyroid ima artery is present in less than 10% of individuals. It can arise from the brachiocephalic trunk, the aortic arch, or the common carotid or subclavian arteries and it enters the lower part of the isthmus.

The inferior thyroid artery travels with the recurrent laryngeal nerve, and the superior thyroid artery travels with the external laryngeal nerve. These are important relations to remember in removing part/all of the thyroid gland when the arteries must be tied off. Damage to the nerves results in a weak and hoarse voice.

The superior and middle thyroid veins join the internal jugular vein. The inferior thyroid veins drain to the left brachiocephalic vein (usually).

Parathyroid glands
The parathyroid glands are four small glands, two on each side, lying external to the posterior surface of the thyroid capsule. They are variable in their location, but are generally found above and below the entrance of the inferior thyroid arteries. They are important in the regulation of calcium metabolism. Their variable position can result in damage or removal during thyroid surgery.

Blood supply to the parathyroid glands
The upper and lower parathyroid glands are supplied by the inferior thyroid artery. Small veins join the thyroid veins.

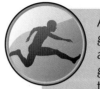

As many as 50% of thyroid glands have a pyramidal lobe, a superior extension of the gland that is usually seen near the isthmus. The pyramidal lobe represents a remnant of the thyroglossal duct, a tube by which the gland is connected to the foramen cecum in the embryo during its descent from the tongue into the neck.

- List the individual bones of which the skull is composed.
- List the openings in the base of the skull and their main contents.
- Describe the anatomy of the scalp, including its blood and nerve supply.
- Define the areas of the face supplied by the divisions of the trigeminal nerve.
- Describe the anatomy of the dura mater and its reflections.
- Describe the anatomy of the cavernous sinus and its contents.
- List the parts of the brain and describe their relationship to the dural folds and the anterior, middle, and posterior cranial cavities.
- Describe the formation of the arterial circle of Willis and its relationship to the main arteries of the brain.
- Describe the origin, function, and circulation of cerebrospinal fluid.
- List the cranial nerves and their functions.
- Describe the course of CN V in the cranial cavity and the route and destination of its branches.
- Describe the course of CN VII in the cranial cavity and the route and destination of its branches.
- Describe the boundaries and contents of the orbital cavity.
- Discuss the actions of the muscles of the eye.
- Describe the anatomy of the parotid gland and the structures passing through it.
- Discuss the boundaries and contents of the infratemporal fossa.
- Describe the boundaries and contents of the pterygopalatine fossa.
- Describe the temporomandibular joint.
- List the branches of the mandibular nerve and what they supply.
- Describe the walls surrounding the tympanic cavity and its contents.
- Outline the components of the internal ear.
- Describe the deep cervical fascia of the neck.
- Describe the boundaries and contents of the posterior triangle.
- Outline the cervical plexus.
- What muscles are classed as suprahyoid, and what is their nerve supply?
- What is the blood and nerve supply of the pharynx?
- Outline the walls of the nasal cavity.
- Discuss the nerve supply of the tongue.
- Describe the laryngeal membranes.
- Describe the internal anatomy of the larynx.
- List the actions and nerve supply of the intrinsic muscles of the larynx.
- Describe the muscles that affect the tension of the vocal folds and width of the rima glottidis.
- Describe the parasympathetic ganglia in the head, their location, and the nerves associated with each.

Index

Specific arteries, muscles, nerves, and veins are listed under their individual names, not grouped under general entries.

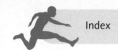

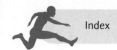

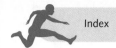

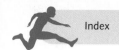

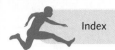

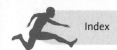

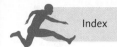

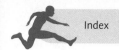

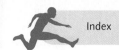

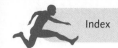

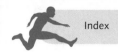

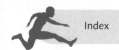